The ethics of survivor research

Guidelines for the ethical conduct of research carried out by mental health service users and survivors

Alison Faulkner

First published in Great Britain in November 2004 by

The Policy Press
Fourth Floor, Beacon House
Queen's Road
Bristol BS8 1QU
UK

Tel no +44 (0)117 331 4054
Fax no +44 (0)117 331 4093
E-mail tpp-info@bristol.ac.uk
www.policypress.org.uk

© Alison Faulkner 2004
All illustrations © Angela Martin

Published for the Joseph Rowntree Foundation by The Policy Press

ISBN 1 86134 641 7

British Library Cataloguing in Publication Data
A catalogue record for this report is available from the British Library.

Library of Congress Cataloging-in-Publication Data
A catalog record for this report has been requested.

Alison Faulkner is an Independent Survivor Researcher.

The **Joseph Rowntree Foundation** has supported this project as part of its programme of research and innovative development projects, which it hopes will be of value to policy makers, practitioners and service users. The facts presented and views expressed in this report are, however, those of the author and not necessarily those of the Foundation.

The statements and opinions contained within this publication are solely those of the author and not of The University of Bristol or The Policy Press. The University of Bristol and The Policy Press disclaim responsibility for any injury to persons or property resulting from any material published in this publication.

The Policy Press works to counter discrimination on grounds of gender, race, disability, age and sexuality.

Cover design by Qube Design Associates, Bristol
Printed in Great Britain by Hobbs the Printers Ltd, Southampton

Contents

Acknowledgements

Grateful thanks go to all those people who took part in this research, and gave of their considerable experience in the interests of helping others. Particular thanks go to Viv Lindow, who developed and initiated this project and gave support and assistance throughout. Thanks also to Vida Field for transcribing the tapes and for our many discussions about their content; and to Premila Trivedi for our discussions over tea about ethics and for cofacilitating the focus group with black participants. Many thanks go to the advisory group (see Appendix C) for their helpful guidance throughout the project and their comments on the report as it progressed. And, finally, thanks to Lesley Jones and Emma Stone for their supportive guidance from the Joseph Rowntree Foundation.

Acronyms and abbreviations

ARW	Advocacy Really Works (organisation run by Roberta Wetherell and Andrew Wetherell)
COREC	Central Office for Research Ethics Committees
ECT	electroconvulsive therapy
MHF	Mental Health Foundation
NICE	National Institute for Clinical Excellence
REC	Research Ethics Committee
TCPS	Trans-Cultural Psychiatry Society
TRUE	Training in Research skills for service Users: project Evaluation (collaborative research project funded by INVOLVE)
UFM	User Focused Monitoring (programme of work based at the Sainsbury Centre for Mental Health)

Executive summary

These guidelines are intended to assist researchers, trainers in research skills and interviewers working from the perspective of mental health service users and survivors. They are intended as helpful guidance on the ethical issues to be considered prior to the design and conduct of any survivor research project or research training programme. While the focus of these guidelines is on 'survivor research' or user-led research, they have significant implications for the involvement of service users in research initiated by academic and other researchers.

Based on consultation with around 50 service user and survivor researchers through questionnaires, individual interviews and focus groups around the UK, the guidelines present helpful suggestions and checklists, as well as quotations reflecting the experience of those consulted, and reference to further resources.

The guidelines are intended for mental health service user/survivor researchers, trainers and interviewers engaged in:

- survivor research, user-controlled research, user-led research;
- research involving service users;
- service monitoring and evaluation;
- training in research or related skills;

as well as for service user/survivor groups and organisations intending to commission or carry out research. The guidelines are also useful for academic researchers looking to involve service users in their research activity in line with the *Research Governance Framework for Health and Social Care* (DH, 2001), any researchers working in the mental health field, Research Ethics Committees and NHS Research and Development Committees.

The guidelines follow the progress of a research project:

1. Underlying principles
   Clarity and transparency; empowerment; identity; commitment to change; respect; equal opportunities; theoretical approach; accountability.
2. Planning and design
   Being involved from the start; adequate funding; negotiating access; flexibility; Ethics Committees; dissemination and feedback.
3. Recruitment and involvement (of fellow researchers)
   Recruitment; inclusivity; payment; other incentives.
4. Training, support and supervision
   Training; support and supervision; researcher safety.
5. Involving participants
   Confidentiality; informed consent; support for participants; payment to participants.
6. Analysis and feedback
   Analysis and interpretation; feedback to participants.
7. Dissemination and implementation
   Dissemination; implementation of research; case study: the Somerset Spirituality Project.
8. Research Ethics Committees.

"Survivor research should attempt to counter the stigma and discrimination experienced by survivors in society."

The issues addressed by these ethical guidelines differ from other similar guidelines in the research field in that they focus on being and working with mental health service users throughout the research process. This has implications for many areas of research, from the principles underlying the research (such as empowerment, respect, clarity and transparency) through the conduct of the research, support and training to dissemination and implementation. One key issue is the value of being involved from the very start of a project – just as relevant for user involvement in research as it is for user-led research. Another is the importance of flexibility throughout the research process, in order to reflect the different needs and abilities of co-researchers and interviewers and the extra time needed sometimes to deal with distress experienced along the way.

> "There needs to be some more flexibility but on the other hand we want to be able to work properly. That takes some help and training and that bit of extra support."

The guidelines also give considerable emphasis to giving feedback to participants, dissemination to local and relevant stakeholders, and a commitment to change or action based on research findings. These reflect people's concern about treating participants with respect, the potential for empowerment and the role of research within people's lives.

The guidelines examine the role of training in research skills for mental health service users and survivors, with suggestions for further reading and guidance on effective training. The same section (4) examines the importance of providing support and supervision to service users engaged in research, and recommends separating 'support' into separate functions in order to ensure that appropriate support is in place:

• emotional support (for example, peer support, debriefing);

• practical support (for example, administration, finance, travel);

• research-related support (for example, supervision to team or to project coordinator).

> "One of the criteria we came up with is that all those involved in a project, including the coordinator, should have access to support and supervision and this should be set up at the beginning."

Crucially, the issue of payment is addressed in these guidelines, both for research participants and for service users working as researchers and interviewers. While the guidelines suggest that people should be paid real money for real work, there are circumstances in which this is difficult and individual choice should be respected. Resources offering advice and guidance on paying people who are on benefits are referenced.

In the mental health field in particular, there has been a considerable increase in both local and national research projects and initiatives involving or led by service users and survivors. Government policy has encouraged this through the *Research Governance Framework* (DH, 2001), which advocates consumer involvement in all stages of the research process. Consequently, many research funders are calling for academic research to involve consumers as a condition of funding. There is a distinction to be made between survivor-controlled research and 'user or consumer involvement in research', and the focus of these guidelines is on the former. However, many of the ethical issues are similar, making the guidelines valuable in the support of the *Research Governance Framework*.

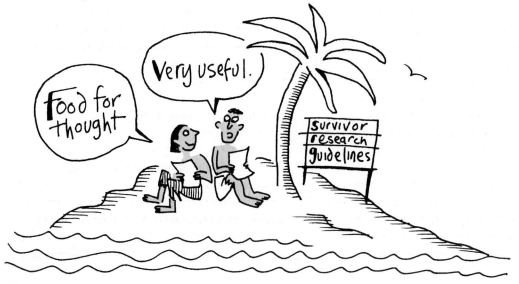

©Angela Martin

Introduction

These guidelines are based on the research reported in Appendix A and on the experience and expertise of many other survivor and professional research groups and organisations. They are not intended as rules, but rather as guidance on issues to be considered prior to the design and conduct of any survivor research project or research training programme. In some cases a particular view is given by the author on behalf of the research undertaken, but in other cases it is made clear that the issue in question needs to be discussed and decided by the research team or individual researcher(s) involved.

The guidelines follow the progress of the research cycle: beginning with underlying principles and finishing with the implementation of results and recommendations.

What is survivor research?

It seems sensible to start by identifying what is meant by 'survivor research' in order that we can be clear about whom these guidelines are intended for. The growth of both national and local survivor research projects has been very rapid during the past few years, with some attendant concerns about quality and standards. There are many different forms of what may be called survivor research, user-led or user-controlled research, and a great many more forms of 'user involvement in research' where the control of the research does not lie with service users or survivors. While these guidelines are primarily intended for the former, that is, research being carried out from a mental health service user/survivor perspective, they are also relevant for people involved in the latter, since many of the issues are universal and pertinent to conduct of good practice anywhere in the mental health field.

However, there may well be different levels of *power* within these different manifestations of user/survivor research, depending on who is funding and managing the research, and this will influence the degree to which user/survivor researchers can determine the direction of the research and the way in which it can be carried out.

The Mental Health Foundation's Strategies for Living programme has come up with a broad definition of user-led (or survivor) research, as follows:

> In the work of Strategies for Living we mean research in which service users or survivors select the topics for research; are members of the steering group; design the research project; ideally, are the researchers and interviewers or have professional researchers as allies; and have control over the funding. User-led research for us also means ongoing appropriate training and support, including peer support; recognising that the process is important as well as the product; sharing findings in relevant ways to relevant audiences, especially other service users; informing services and service development; and informing participants about the results and any action. (Nicholls et al, 2003)

Members of different parts of the Strategies for Living programme were consulted during the formation of the present guidelines.

Similarly, the Sainsbury Centre for Mental Health has developed a nationwide *User Focused Monitoring* (UFM) network that provides support for service users who want to become or who are involved in monitoring their own local services. They have recently established a set of criteria for what constitutes a UFM project (UFM Network,

2003). Again, several members of UFM projects were consulted in the formation of these guidelines.

Finally, it may be helpful here to explore the terms 'survivor' and 'service user'. They can be used rather differently by different people, but (as in the earlier example of UFM projects) the term 'service user' is usually used where the people to be involved in a project are using or have used mental health services. Very often, in the context of research, this means they have used the service being explored within the research project. (Different definitions of mental health services may be used; for example, some people will refer only to secondary mental health services, others will include the use of talking treatments and primary mental health care support.) The term 'survivor' is often intended as a more broad term to include people who have experienced mental or emotional distress, whether or not they have used mental health services. However, 'survivor' may also be used politically to refer to people who have survived mental health services and/or treatments; in this sense it is shorthand for 'psychiatric system survivor'.

In summary these guidelines are intended for:

- Service user/survivor researchers, trainers and interviewers engaged in:
  - survivor research, user-controlled research, user-led research;
  - research involving service users;
  - service monitoring and evaluation;
  - training in research or related skills.
- Service user/survivor groups and organisations intending to commission or carry out research.

These guidelines are useful for:

- academic (non-survivor) researchers looking to involve service users in their research activity;
- any researchers working in the mental health field;
- Research Ethics Committees (RECs);
- NHS Research and Development Committees.

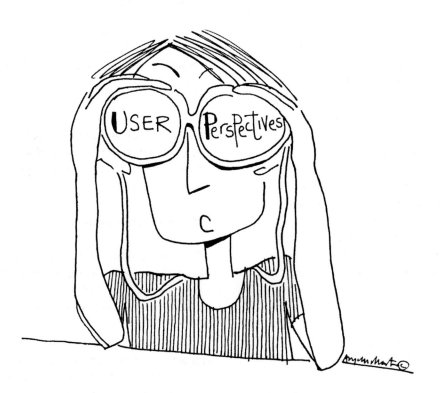

Underlying principles

The principles underlying a research programme or individual project are worth exploring in order for all participants to be clear about the nature of the research and the approach to be adopted from the start. These principles may be underlying or unstated aims of the research – such as the empowerment of mental health service users, or the adoption of an agenda for change. On the other hand, an underlying principle might represent a theoretical approach to research in general (such as a belief in knowledge for its own sake) or to an individual project in particular.

In the research carried out for these guidelines, there was considerable consensus of opinion about the underlying principles presented to participants: service user empowerment, equal opportunities, respect for all those involved, and the rights of researchers and participants. People also suggested other principles for inclusion: a commitment to change being the most notable.

It is notable that many principles proposed by survivor researchers have emerged out of the experience of being researched; some difficult experiences at the receiving end of mainstream researchers have led to people wishing to undertake a different approach to their own research.

Clarity and transparency

A clear and open approach towards all of the people involved in a project, co-researchers and research participants in particular, can avoid many problems further down the line. There are many examples throughout the process of research that demonstrate the importance of this principle. For example, it is vital to be open about the pay-offs for being involved in a project and about any

potential difficulties or risks, and to let people know about the approach you are taking towards recruitment and training (see Chapters 4 and 5). It is also vital to be open about your confidentiality policy with participants, and to tell a participant if you plan to breach confidentiality with them (see Chapter 6). Clarity and transparency can be seen to underlie many of the other issues covered in these guidelines.

Empowerment

Most of the people involved in the research for these guidelines were of the view that survivor research should aim for or facilitate the empowerment of service users, although several felt the need to clarify what this means:

> "If empowerment means making it possible for people to challenge their lack of power, gain more personal power and power politically, then it is crucial."

> "If it means giving power back.... "

> "The more control you have over research the more chance it will be empowering and you will find you have benefited. If you don't have any control then the more chance you will find it harmful."

In practical terms, empowerment means adopting an agenda for change (see later in this chapter), ensuring that service users' voices are heard through the research, and challenging attitudes about people with a mental illness diagnosis. It also has significant implications for the way in which research participants are treated and involved during the research process (see Chapter 6). Empowerment was raised as being particularly significant for black and minority ethnic communities and for people held in secure provision:

> "[Interviewing in forensic services] shows the interviewers that they can produce valuable work that will change services and shows those in the units they can have a say in services and make a change. They're more likely to start speaking out if you get those results. This promotes user empowerment."

This principle clearly links survivor research with *emancipatory research*, that is, research that has empowerment at its heart. Emancipatory research was described by Barnes and Mercer (1997) as enabling (as against disabling), reflexive and self-critical. By enabling, they mean that research participants should be enabled by the research to have a voice in their own lives. By reflexive, they suggest that researchers should reflect upon their role in the research process, acknowledging their own identity and power within it. In a chapter in the same book, Beresford and Wallcraft (1997) refer to it as follows:

> Undertaking emancipatory research has been part of the survivor movement's project of survivors speaking and acting for themselves; improving their lives and liberating themselves from an oppressive psychiatric system; of changing and equalising relationships between research and research subjects, and developing survivors' own knowledge collectively.

Identity

In assuming what is meant by 'survivor research', the issue of identity is perhaps in danger of being overlooked. However a number of interviewees raised it as a fundamental issue needing to be clarified from the start of a research project. It is a principle of emancipatory research that the power relationships that exist between the researcher and the researched are challenged through process and through participation. As mentioned earlier (What is survivor research?, p 1), survivor research is research that is carried out from a mental health service user or survivor perspective. It is possible that research coordinators or trainers may not be survivors or service users, but that the work is being directed by people who do identify themselves in this way. Either way this shared identity between

the researchers and the researched is a vital element of survivor research.

Researchers may need to debate what is meant by a 'service user' or 'survivor' at the start of a project; for the UFM criteria, a definition of service user was settled on one that includes "people who have used or currently use mental health services". This is due to their primary focus on the people who are or who have been in receipt of the services under evaluation. In the case of work in forensic services or other specific service areas, the project participants may need to discuss whether or to what extent users of that particular service are to be involved in the research.

A further issue concerning identity is the value placed on identifying yourself as a service user or survivor – and finding a comfortable means of doing so – when introducing yourself to research participants. Many survivor researchers have found that it makes a positive difference to interviewees to be interviewed by a fellow service user or survivor (see Faulkner and Layzell, 2000; Rose, 2001).

Commitment to change

A vital component of the potential for research to facilitate empowerment lies in its commitment to change. In the questionnaire, several people added this to the section on underlying principles; and in the interviews, many talked about the importance of research leading to change and not to knowledge for its own sake.

Among the proponents of an agenda for change were the representatives of UFM (UFM Network, 2003), whose criteria state:

The aims of the research are to:

- evaluate existing services for people with mental health problems; and to
- make positive changes in mental health services and generate creative alternatives to existing services.

Change was also seen as particularly significant for minority groups and marginalised groups whose voices may not often be heard through research.

"Participation is affected if people don't see a prospect of change. Especially for black service users, who start off with issues about engagement in services anyway. The issue of change is one reason why black people can be reluctant to get involved in research."

Starting research with an agenda for change may not always be sufficient for individual researchers or even research teams to be able to implement their results and bring about change; further discussion of this issue is to be found in Chapter 8. Also, where research is breaking new ground in relation to survivor knowledge, it may not lead to immediate change but may be contributing to a change in views or attitudes. As one person said, it can be that we:

"undertake research not with the certainty that it could lead to the kind of change that survivors might want, but with that goal in mind."

Respect

Respect, it would seem, is an easy principle to agree with but less easy to define in practical terms. People who discussed this principle in the interviews often referred to the importance of respecting people and their right to express their views, within the context of involving a group of service users in a research project. This would be something they would address in the training, in order that everyone involved might respect each other's views. It is equally important to respect the views of the people who are participating in the research, whether as interviewees, focus group members or questionnaire respondents. This means ensuring that they are listened to and their views recorded fully and, further, that the training given to interviewers emphasises the importance of these issues.

Respect was raised specifically in relation to research in a forensic setting: that it is important to respect the individual using the service, and their rights to comment on those services, regardless of what they may have done to merit detention in this setting.

Equal opportunities

Several people referred to respect within the context of principles of equal opportunities and diversity: that we all need to be aware of the potential for oppressive language or behaviour. Within the forensic services, it was emphasised that all views need to be represented, because:

"Often the quiet people don't get heard."

To this end, the researcher stated her commitment to matching interviewers with interviewees on race, sex and sexuality where appropriate. Similarly, the UFM (2003) guide states:

Projects should actively aim to secure the participation [as researchers, interviewees and wider contributors] of a large proportion of service users who have used the services under evaluation, including those people whose voices are rarely heard.

Several people raised the importance of hearing from people on the margins of service use: from homeless people, from people of different ages within black and minority ethnic communities, and people with a myriad of 'overlapping' identities:

"I am concerned about overlapping identities so people with learning disabilities, deaf people who are also survivors will have few opportunities to be involved as researchers."

As this last quotation illustrates, there are (at least) two different aspects to be considered: equal opportunities in relation to the research project (content) and equal opportunities in relation to the research process. The research therefore needs to think about the ways in which the views of diverse communities are part of the project from the start, including the co-researchers and interviewers as well as research participants. If we are committed to breaking down the barriers between the researchers and the researched, then it is vital that we are addressing these issues from the start.

Theoretical approach

The value of being clear and transparent about the theoretical approach you are adopting in research is that people can make a genuine judgement about whether to become involved or not, whether as participant, co-researcher or interviewer.

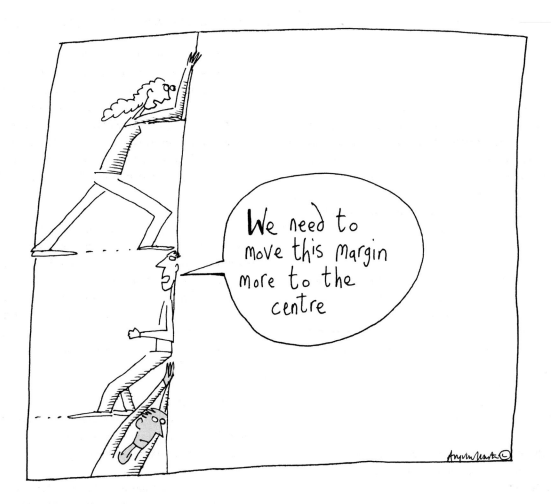

In the development of these guidelines, it was members of black and minority ethnic communities who most supported the importance of transparency about the theoretical underpinnings of research. The Mind/Trans-Cultural Psychiatry Society guidelines for ethical mental health research involving issues of race, ethnicity and culture (Patel, 1999) are the only other ethical guidelines found by this author which address this issue:

> Researchers should critique and make explicit the theories and theoretical concepts used in their research, examining their validity and reliability in relation to the population that is to be studied. (p 15)

Many such values emerged out of past experiences, and this was no exception. People felt that black communities have in the past been damaged by research carried out on them which was fundamentally incompatible with their own beliefs about mental illness and/or about the dominance of racism and oppression within society. Hence the importance of transparency, or honesty about the theoretical approach being adopted in any research, particularly in survivor research. In

survivor research we would contend that our theoretical perspective is central to the principle of empowerment; the traditional view of research as 'objective' is not shared since all research has its own perspective, which therefore omits others. For example, research undertaken from a clinical medical perspective is likely to omit significant social issues.

Similar issues were touched on by other people involved in the development of these guidelines, in relation to (challenging) the dominance of the medical model in mainstream research, and in the interests of the principle of transparency – both to potential co-researchers and to research participants. Furthermore, the questionnaire item "Researchers to make explicit any underlying beliefs or theories" received agreement from 14 out of the 15 respondents, reinforcing this approach.

Accountability to ...

i) Society

In the interests of comparability with other professional guidelines for the conduct of research, the issue of accountability to society was addressed in the development of these guidelines. This issue, along with other principles of accountability, provoked a range of responses. For some people, it was interpreted as ensuring research is socially inclusive and diverse, so there was no conflict here with a principle addressing equal opportunities.

However, several people raised difficulties with the idea of being accountable to society, on the basis that society is not accountable to mental health service users: that responsibility (accountability) confers some rights and mental health service users do not currently have equal rights within society. Comments included:

> "Do they have responsibility to us?"

> "Is there a possibility that our allegiance to society might conflict with our allegiance to survivors?"

Still other people consulted emphasised the fact that we, as survivors, are members of society and that divisions or conflicts should not be created or strengthened.

> "Research should raise the profile of mental health and distress in society, should counter the stigma and discrimination based on a diagnosis. It should be relevant to a wider society because everyone at some point experiences mental distress and we have a responsibility to make people aware of that."

> "Survivor research should attempt to counter the stigma and discrimination experienced by survivors in society."

Politically, research is deemed to be accountable to society through such frameworks as the *Research Governance Framework*, which emphasises the role of public involvement in research.

Perhaps, then, the conclusion of the present research is to suggest that researchers reflect on this issue, and aim to clarify the relationship between their proposed research and 'society at large'.

ii) Service user movement/communities/groups

In the questionnaire, the issue of accountability to service user and survivor communities raised considerable variation in response. Nine people out of the 15 responded in the affirmative to the question "Do you believe that survivor research needs to have responsibilities towards relevant mental health service user groups, communities and individuals?", three responded "No" and three "Not sure".

This range of responses was elaborated in the interviews to reflect the difficulty of being responsible or accountable to *all* service users/survivors. A researcher might have difficulty designing a project to reflect the concerns of the 'wider service user community' on the grounds that the latter is too diverse in itself for every research project to be of concern. The prospect of determining some kind of consensus of priorities for survivor research did not seem feasible or reasonable. This was also raised by black interviewees as a potential barrier to research that might be of relevance to black and minority ethnic user and survivor communities.

An aspect of accountability that attracted more support was the value of accountability to local communities and to local service user groups in particular. The UFM (2003) guide specifies local communities and local issues as their core concern: "*Where we've pitched our tent is on local issues*" (italics for emphasis). The strength of this approach is ensuring that the service evaluated is of concern to local service users and that local people are involved throughout the process.

Another view expressed in the interviews was that we *do* need to be accountable to the broader service user community or communities. Some argued for a "*formal and structured responsibility to survivor groups*": for mechanisms to be in place to ensure that there is evidence from the grassroots of service user groups to support the need and value of a piece of research.

> "Yes we should have responsibility to other survivors; it's all about responsibility to survivors ... commitment to social justice for users, survivors. We have a responsibility to make sure people get their voices heard in the way they want them to be heard."

So, it would seem that we need to be quite sophisticated in our understanding of what it means to be accountable to service users and survivors. The elements within the questionnaire on this issue that evoked most agreement were as follows:

- the impact of research to be meaningful to user/ survivor groups and communities;
- research not to perpetuate stereotypes of people with mental health problems;
- researchers to make explicit any underlying beliefs or theories;
- research to be of high quality;
- results of research to be disseminated in accessible formats.

Protection from harm: *a note*

The principle of 'protection from harm' is included in most professional guidelines for the ethical conduct of research. It is also an issue deemed to be of high importance in RECs when considering new research proposals. It was not an issue that attracted a great deal of interest in this research. Although generally signed up to in the questionnaire, it was also of concern to some people that protection of mental health service users from harm can at times be patronising and inappropriate. As a couple of people said, people can be distressed by an interview and can nevertheless wish to continue and to contribute. Distress is not necessarily equivalent to harm.

Suggestions for underlying principles

- Talk about the principles with which you are approaching your research at the start. Consider such issues as:
  - empowerment
  - identity
  - commitment to change
  - respect
  - equal opportunities.
- Be as clear and transparent as you can be about the research and everyone's role within it, about the incentives and risks for both participants and co-researchers and about the theoretical approach underlying the research.
- Consider to what extent your research is accountable to society, and/or to mental health service users and survivors both locally and nationally.

"In a palliative care project people got upset but it was positive for them. Becoming distressed is not the same as harm. There must be routes for follow-up. It's not an excuse for going round upsetting people.... "

We address this issue in more detail in the chapter on involving participants (Chapter 6), within the context of endeavouring to ensure that people have support to deal with any distress caused by an interview. However, it is worth pointing out that people within mental health services rarely have the opportunity to speak for an hour about themselves or to tell their story, and this in itself can often be a positive experience.

"Nobody has ever sort of asked my opinion on anything like this before, you know - how I feel about anything. It's all within the psychiatrist's room, and you have to agree with what he says, and that's it, sort of thing (quoted in Faulkner and Layzell, 2000)."

3

Planning and design of research

Being involved from the start

A principle raised by several people was the importance of being involved from the start of a project. Despite being survivor research and hence under the control of survivor researchers, it cannot be assumed that those people who need to be are indeed involved from the very start of a project. This might apply to co-researchers and interviewers who are brought in somewhere down the line, and who subsequently wish to make changes to plans or conditions established before they were involved.

> "Everyone who is going to be involved should be involved right from the beginning … I wasn't involved in the talk at the beginning so I didn't know much about it so I felt I'd been asked to do this piece of work but I'd been left in the dark, getting messages passed to me but never having any proper meetings with anyone."

This may not always be possible to achieve for practical reasons. If you are not able to involve everyone from the start, it is vital that you are clear about why this was and about what it is possible to influence or to change about the project.

Adequate funding

Planning for flexibility has implications for funding and for other resources too. It is vital that these issues are thought through at an early stage, in order that the most is made of what resources may be available to a project. Additional elements that might need to go into a funding application are given in the following suggested checklist. Please do not regard this as a list of essentials; it is a list of suggestions that may help you to plan your project and to be prepared for things that you may otherwise overlook.

Suggested checklist for funding

- support for co-researchers and interviewers (may be an additional support worker or alternative);
- external supervision, for example, to coordinator of a project;
- enough funding to include more people than the project needs, to cover for periods of absence;
- physical resources, such as space and communication technology;
- training;
- social events/time to meet with each other;
- dissemination: in different formats relevant to your project (for example, language, accessible, written and oral presentations);
- insurance – liability;
- fees for participants;
- payment to researchers.

Negotiating access

Many research projects can fall at this early hurdle. Access to a service may need to be negotiated, and subsequently access to individual participants may have to be negotiated as well. In some projects, professionals may act as the gatekeepers to patients, and this may present difficulties but it may also be the only ethical way to proceed. For example, in one project on risk, the researchers did not wish to know the names of people who were considered to be at risk of causing harm before they had consented to take part in the project. Consequently, the research was presented to patients by the staff. In another project, researchers were concerned that staff only allowed them access to patients who they considered to be 'well enough' to take part. The need to depend on professional gatekeepers may also be a problem where they are busy and may not support the research, or act protectively of patients when researchers do not feel it is appropriate to do so.

A couple of researchers emphasised the importance of having a key member of staff in support of the research; this may be someone with the status to enforce issues of access or it may be someone closer to the patients or service users who can help in practical ways.

Flexibility

Flexibility might almost be a key underlying principle. It is a quality that seems to be essential for survivor research and also to any research involving service users or consumers initiated by (non-survivor) academic researchers. Flexibility needs to be planned in from the start of any project, both in terms of timescales and deadlines, and in terms of resources to allow for people becoming distressed or unwell during the project or needing extra support.

For a successful research marathon, flex your timescales, deadlines and resources

Build in time pockets

RESEARCH Marathon

Flexibility was emphasised by those people who were coordinating large programmes of survivor research, perhaps because of their overall responsibility for seeing the individual projects through to the end. It was also emphasised in situations where survivors did not have overall control over the deadlines or outputs for the research. Some suggestions for managing flexibility are as follows:

- at the planning stage, build in more time at the end of the project in order to plan for unforeseen eventualities;
- reschedule the timetable and reducing the scope of the research;
- build support in from the start (see Chapter 5).

Flexibility needs to have boundaries too, as a couple of people pointed out. Endless flexibility might mean that a project does not get completed:

"There needs to be some more flexibility but on the other hand we want to be able to work properly. That takes some help and training and that bit of extra support."

Ethics Committees

Research Ethics Committees are dealt with in more detail in Chapter 9. However, research access to many services within the NHS cannot be achieved without getting approval from the local REC first. This, therefore, needs to be included in the plan for your research project, and the timing adjusted accordingly. RECs meet on a regular basis, but you do need to find out how often and when in order to cause as little delay as possible to the progress of your project.

Dissemination and feedback

Although you are only at the start of your project, it is important to think through to the end when you are planning it. As outlined in Chapters 7 and 8, dissemination and feedback are very important issues to survivor researchers and participants. This involves both time and money, and therefore needs to be planned in from the start: there needs to be enough time at the end to disseminate the work to the relevant stakeholders and practitioners or policy makers, as well as time and resources to feed back results to your research participants. There is more detail on this subject in Chapter 7.

Suggestions for planning and design

- Ideally, everyone should be involved from the start of the research. If this is not possible, it is vital that you are clear about why this was and about what it is possible to influence or to change about the project.
- A budget checklist is given on page 9.
- Access to research participants and services may need to be negotiated at an early stage. While the need to rely on professional gatekeepers may raise problems, it may also be an asset to negotiate with someone who can offer support from within the service.
- The potential for flexibility needs to be built in from the start: issues such as support, rescheduling the timetable or scope of the research and anticipating the need for extra time at the end of the project, may need to be considered.
- Find out if your project needs to have the approval of your local REC; this will require extra time and resources to negotiate.
- Plan in some time and resources for the dissemination of your findings and feedback to research participants.

Additional resources on planning and design

- College of Occupational Therapists (September 2003) *Research ethics guidelines*, London: College of Occupational Therapists.
- Nicholls, V. et al (1999) *The DIY guide to survivor research*, London: Mental Health Foundation.

4

Recruitment and involvement

This chapter is concerned with the involvement of people (mental health service users and survivors) in *carrying out* the research, whether as co-researchers, interviewers or advisers to the project. Chapter 6 looks at the involvement of participants in the research process.

Recruitment

We include this in the event that project coordinators or researchers are seeking to involve more or local service users – or those using a particular service – in a new project. This is an area where clarity and transparency are essential to potential recruits. It is important to be clear about how many people you wish to involve, and not to become carried away with the enthusiasm of a large group of people, involve too many and find out further down the line that there are insufficient resources to support them. Equally, you may wish to include rather more people than you need in order to manage periods of absence. Either way, it is helpful to think this through before the start of the recruitment.

Two projects with experience of this are the User Focused Monitoring (UFM) project, which recruits extensively in local communities, and Advocacy Really Works (ARW), working in forensic services. Generally, the latter do not recruit people who have used forensic services themselves, but those who have used other mental health services. In this instance, because of some of the difficulties and constraints on working in secure settings, it is the policy of ARW to turn down people if they do not feel that they are ready for the work following the training.

"Because we are recruiting people from acute and community services who haven't had experience of forensic services, there are two important factors: why they are doing it and training so that they can understand the differences, because there really is a difference. So we do quite an extensive training programme and then give them the option to opt out at the end. We also tell them there is an option for us to not use them."

UFM projects, on the other hand, recruit people locally from a variety of settings and adopt a policy of 'inclusivity' (see below). They contact service user groups, reaching out to people in the specific services being evaluated; some have used radio, posters and visits to local agencies (for example, those dealing with black and minority ethnic communities, homeless people or people who have experienced domestic violence). In some instances people have talked face to face with service users and news is spread by word of mouth.

A final note on involving people in research: different skills and experience may be relevant in different settings. It was pointed out by ARW that care needs to be taken over matching interviewers with service user interviewees, for example, not sending mothers of young children to interview in a sex offender unit. The same may be true for other settings or for individuals working within certain settings.

Inclusivity

A key issue for new projects is whether or not you intend to establish criteria, assess and 'pass' or 'fail' people for involvement in a project, whether before or after training. This is something that must be made clear from the start. It is a sensitive issue and will need to be handled with care and respect, but it is vital to be clear about your intentions.

Generally speaking, the people consulted in the development of these guidelines were in favour of inclusivity, that is, including as many people as possible who come forward to take part in the research process, recognising people's different skills and their potential for contributing in different ways.

> "We like to involve as many people as possible – be inclusive, find a role for anybody but that does need time and money."

Some people may not wish to take part in interviewing but may be able to contribute to the design of questions and ideas for topics; equally, others may prefer office work to taking an active role in the interviewing. Some of the discussion around this issue concerned the importance of maintaining the quality of the research amid concern for participants; hence the need on occasions to suggest to individuals that they may not be ready to take part in interviewing.

As pointed out earlier in this section, the projects going into forensic services felt the need to be more cautious about who can be included in the interviewing process. UFM projects have used the group process and supervision to manage their inclusive approach; individuals can watch others, and play another role until they are ready to become fully involved. They too occasionally need to suggest to individuals that they may not be ready to interview others.

> "A lot of projects have tended to work by not setting very formal criteria for becoming involved, partly because they don't want to put people off who feel they don't have the confidence, the ability, the skills.... Being so open, however, has become an issue on some projects and I think the way that has been dealt with is by ensuring access to some sort of supervision within the group process."

Payment for involvement

Payments available for co-researchers and interviewers can be an influence on your recruitment policy; if the equivalent of a salary payment is to be offered then there is likely to be a more rigorous recruitment policy.

> "People should be appropriately and equally paid for their contributions. Contributions can

be different so we identified different rates of payment according to what you are doing."

Most people were in favour of real payment for real work: for co-researchers and interviewers to be paid a reasonable daily rate or sessional rate for the work being done. However, some did point out the need for flexibility in this, due to some people being on state welfare benefits and unable to receive more than a set amount per week. Another issue raised was that some people prefer not to accept payment because they prefer to be volunteers. This preference should be respected. The emphasis should be on choice; it may be possible to spread payments over several weeks in order to ensure that people are not being paid more than their permitted allowance, or to offer people tokens or vouchers in place of cash[1].

> "There is an issue that some people do not want to be paid and they should not be obliged to be paid but then that money can go to the organisation or to an organisation of their choice.... Payment may not be possible always, there has to be flexibility. But in principle we would want to be raising these issues as a priority."

However, the issue of payment does bring into play the relationship between rewards and responsibilities; if you are being paid a proper rate for the work, then the work/employer can have more formal expectations of you, possibly even a formal contract. This may be a good thing in some circumstances and not in others.

Either way, several people raised the need for people involved in a project to be given advice and information about permitted payments and any potential risk to their current benefits. Some projects have engaged a Benefits Adviser to offer this advice at an early stage.

---

[1] Vouchers have similar implications for tax and benefits to cash, so individuals may need to check this before making their decision.

Sources of information about payments

- Mental Health Foundation (2003) *A fair day's pay: A guide to benefits, service user involvement and payments*, London: Mental Health Foundation (www.mentalhealth.org.uk).
- INVOLVE (2003) 'A guide to paying members of the public who are actively involved in research' (www.invo.org.uk).
- 'Contributing on equal terms: getting involved and the benefits system', Shaping Our Lives, 2004, tel 020 7095 1159
- Hanley, B. et al (2003) *Involving the public in NHS, public health and social care research: Briefing notes for researchers* (2nd edn), Eastleigh: INVOLVE.

Other incentives

Many other incentives to, and benefits from, involvement in research were mentioned. In many ways, why would anyone be involved in a research project if there were not some benefits from doing so? There needs to be some discussion at the start of the project about the potential benefits and incentives available to people, in order that these can be made clear at the beginning and in the recruitment process. These are some of the benefits mentioned during the course of the consultation:

- new skills
- sharing experiences with other participants
- occupation
- sense of purpose
- potential for future employment

- being involved in effecting change
- sense of belonging to a group.

For some people, the experience of being involved in a project was an incentive in itself:

"…just to be able to talk to other people who'd been through similar kinds of problems, I found it amazing. I found it very, very positive just to be able to speak about very personal things in a non-judgemental kind of environment."

Suggestions for recruitment and involvement

- Thinking through the needs of your project at the start, and considering who and how many people you need to be involved, may avoid problems later on. Recruitment of co-researchers can then be focused on appropriate local groups and settings.
- Be clear with people from the start about what skills and experiences are needed, particularly if you intend to establish criteria for involvement.
- People can be involved in and contribute to a project in a variety of ways, so may not all need the same skills. It may be that a principle of inclusivity will override concerns about skills and experience, in which case careful management and supervision may be needed.
- Ideally, real payment should be offered for real work. However some flexibility is needed here: some people may choose not to be paid, and others may need specialist advice if in receipt of benefits.
- There are many possible incentives to taking part that may be considered as part of a project: new skills, sharing experiences, occupation, and the potential for future employment, being involved in a group and in effecting change.

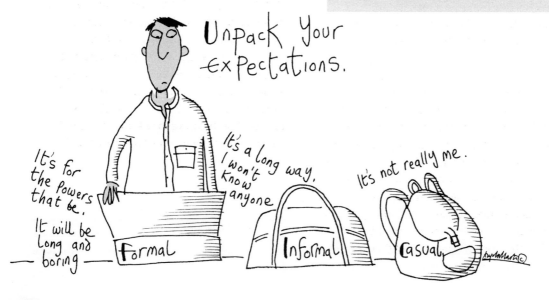

5

Training, support and supervision

Training

Training is an essential element of survivor research, particularly for people who have not done research before, as it is the means by which they will gain skills and knowledge – some key incentives to taking part. All of the people consulted for these guidelines confirmed the significance of good training, with emphasis on support and debriefing, the context of research and issues of accessibility and flexibility. The organisations that have perhaps done the most work on research skills training are the Mental Health Foundation's Strategies for Living programme, the UFM programme at the Sainsbury Centre for Mental Health (neither of which are survivor-led organisations) and ARW (Advocacy Really Works).

It is not the purpose of these guidelines to address training in detail, but rather to look at some of the ethical issues surrounding the delivery of training. Training needs to be accessible and flexible in order to reflect the needs of trainees, as well as preparing people in a responsible manner for what they will be doing and for eventualities along the way. It also needs to be adequate and thorough if it is to ensure high standards of research (see UFM Network, 2003).

One of the aspects raised by interviewees was the timing of training. One group felt quite strongly that training should precede the research for it to be useful, and others felt that it was good practice for training to follow the research process in a step-by-step manner. This may well depend on the time available to carry out a project; if it is to take place over an extended period of time, the training might be better staggered to take place alongside the research rather than risk the possibility that people might forget what they have learnt before having the chance to make use of it.

The elements to be covered in training might include many of the issues covered in these guidelines, as well as the skills required for the relevant research methods to be adopted. Thus, training needs to cover some of the key elements of ethical practice:

- aims and purpose of the research/evaluation
- confidentiality
- informed consent
- support to interviewees
- peer and other support
- risk.

Those whose experience covered working in forensic services emphasised the importance of raising some potentially difficult issues – such as risk and security measures, the range of offences that might have been committed and environmental issues – through training in order to prepare people fully for the nature of the work.

"You have to be realistic which is not easy and be understanding and non-judgemental. You have to raise issues around things like manipulation, because patients in there will manipulate, understandably so because if you are locked up you will do anything to get a bit extra but they are very good at it. It's very difficult. You also have to talk about risk and why there are certain security measures...."

Suggestions for training

- Think about the timing of training and adapt it to the needs of the project and of the trainees.
- Introductory training needs to include some work on the wider context of the project and of research.
- Training needs to be flexible and thorough to adapt to the needs of individuals, and to provide for people with different strengths and levels of experience.
- It is important to think about the context of the training itself: comfortable physical surroundings, refreshments and regular breaks are helpful.
- Training can usefully introduce the aspects of support and supervision, risks and safety measures to be used throughout the project ...
- ... as well as the ways in which participants (or interviewees) will be supported (see below).

Training resources

- Denscombe, M. (1998) *The good research guide for small-scale research projects*, Buckingham: Open University Press.
- Lockey, R. et al (2004) *Training for service user involvement in health and social care research – A study of training provision and participants' experiences (the TRUE Project)*, Worthing: Worthing and Southlands Hospitals NHS Trust.
- Nicholls, V. et al (1999) *The DIY guide to survivor research*, London: Mental Health Foundation.
- Nicholls, V. (2001) *Doing research ourselves*, London: Mental Health Foundation.
- UFM Network (2003) *Doing it for real: A guide to setting up and undertaking a User Focused Monitoring project*, London: Sainsbury Centre for Mental Health (www.scmh.org.uk).

Support and supervision

Many people emphasised the role of both support and supervision, and it was highly rated in the questionnaire. Since these issues are discussed a good deal in connection with survivor research, it seems sensible to attempt to clarify what is meant by them.

"One of the criteria we came up with is that all those involved in a project, including the coordinator, should have access to support and supervision and this should be set up at the beginning."

Support can mean different things to different people, and perhaps what is needed early on in a project is a frank discussion about what people might need in terms of support. It may help to think of it in the following categories:

- emotional support
- practical support
- research-related support.

Emotional support may be needed on an ongoing basis for people who are engaged in work that is distressing and may touch on their own experiences; this is common in survivor research where people are often motivated to become involved because the subject is of personal interest to them/us. This may take the form of regular group/peer support, debriefing after interviews, and possibly additional access to a person whose role it is to support people (as against managing or coordinating the research).

"Maybe there should be another person attached to the project who is not responsible day to day and not focused on the findings. They could concentrate on us and support us."

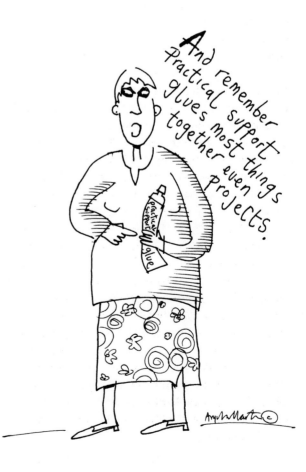

Practical support may be the glue that sticks a project together: money in cash form available for people's expenses, an adequate administrative function, regular communications, travel arrangements or vouchers dealt with, payments available for childcare or other support needs. It cannot be emphasised enough that people need money in advance to pay for things; many people, the author included, have come up against bureaucratic obstacles within organisations that make this difficult. People who are living on benefits are unlikely to be able to buy a rail ticket in advance and wait to be reimbursed. People with physical impairments may have specific needs that will ensure that their participation is equitable.

Research-related support is important to ensure and maintain the standards of the research. This may be in the form of supervision, perhaps to the coordinator of the project or to a whole team. It may be brought in to manage a specific phase, for example the analysis, or may be an ongoing part of the support offered to the project. The nature of supervision may depend on the experience and skills of a coordinator or of the members of a team. Several people emphasised the need for both support and supervision, and an appreciation of the difference between them.

Many people mentioned the importance of managing for the possibility of people becoming unwell and unable to participate in the project for periods of time. This was something that came up within the large group projects in particular: Strategies for Living, UFM and the TRUE Project. All were in agreement that this is something that needs to be managed through advance preparation, flexibility and support. The possibility needs to be planned into the timetable with time and other resources, and it may be possible to introduce extra support at these times. This is one of the areas where flexibility becomes important: perhaps rescheduling the timetable or research process to accommodate people's absences, and/or reducing the scope of the research. Emotional support and the boundaries to that were discussed: the importance of supporting people within the context of the project, but not beyond the boundaries of the relationship. One suggestion was to have some information about people's personal support networks, and to have an agreement about how and when to get in touch with someone on behalf of the person in distress. Another was to develop a crisis plan with team members at the start of the project.

Suggestions for support and supervision

- Think about sources of support and supervision at the start of the project, and their resource implications.
- It may help to break these down into
  - ‣ emotional support
  - ‣ practical support
  - ‣ research-related support/supervision.
- Prepare for the possibility of people needing extra support or being absent from the project due to periods of distress.
- Discuss with team members what seems appropriate in terms of crisis plans or contact with others in the event of distress/absence.
- Time for teambuilding, peer support and fun.

Additional resources on support and supervision

- Faulkner, A. (in press) *Capturing the experiences of those involved in the TRUE Project: A story of colliding worlds*, Eastleigh: INVOLVE (www.invo.org.uk).
- Nicholls, V. et al (2003) *Surviving user-led research: Reflections on supporting user-led research projects*, London: Mental Health Foundation.
- UFM Network (2003) *Doing it for real: A guide to setting up and undertaking a User Focused Monitoring project*, London: Sainsbury Centre for Mental Health (www.scmh.org.uk).

Researcher safety

Researchers do need to give appropriate consideration to the risks that may be involved in a research project, and to introduce reasonable safety measures. The risks may be of physical or of psychological harm to themselves and their colleagues; in addition, managers or employers may be legally responsible in terms of health and safety regulations. These risks apply to any social research endeavour, and particularly to those that involve interviewing in people's own homes where the researcher is unfamiliar with both the interviewee and his or her home and location.

None of us working in the mental health field wishes to be drawn into the stereotypes that exist regarding the association between mental illness diagnoses and violence. Nevertheless, if we know that we are interviewing a group of people who have previously been violent or if we are entering unknown situations, we do need to be prepared for how we might deal with any risks that occur.

One option is for researchers to use a room in a familiar location for interviewing, such as a day centre or other appropriate organisation. This may well have implications for costs, but it does mean that the interviewers can familiarise themselves with the location in advance and that there may be other people around in case of an untoward incident. In addition, it may be appropriate to place oneself nearer the door for the interview and/or to have staff available nearby where interviewing is taking place in certain health or social care settings.

However, this may not be practical and interviewees may prefer to be interviewed in their own homes. There are a number of other safety precautions that may be taken:

- Interview in pairs; if the situation is known to be risky, agree code words to signify ending the interview or other actions.
- Have a mobile phone with you.
- Ensure that someone knows where you are and when. Agree that they ring you at a certain time; *or* agree that the researcher rings the support person when the interview is over; the support person rings the researcher if this has not happened by an agreed time. In this case, both researcher and support person need to have a mobile phone.
- If in any doubt, leave the interview: no research is worth risking your safety.
- In high-risk projects, it may be worth providing de-escalation training to interviewers. ·

It is important to remember that risk is not just about physical harm; some people have experienced psychological or emotional harm through verbal abuse, racism or other offensive language. Similar precautions apply, but it must be emphasised to interviewers that they can leave the interview at any time if they feel that they are at risk of abuse or harm. This also indicates the importance of ensuring appropriate support for interviewers (as discussed earlier): having the opportunity to talk to someone after an interview and having access to peer support can enable interviewers to feel more confident about managing situations.

During the research for these guidelines, one female interviewee told of an experience that proves the need to be properly prepared for this area of work. She interviewed someone alone in a forensic setting when her co-worker did not turn up, and the interviewee disclosed his offence to her which she found very distressing. Training plays a vital role in preparing people for interviewing in high risk situations, as ARW have found:

"We also talk about index offences and what people might have done, which can be horrific but you need to let people know what they're going into. People need to be properly prepared and decide whether they want to do that. We've had occasions when we've had to do a lot of support and downloading when people come out."

Discussion about and preparation for risk is essential; incidents involving potential or actual harm to interviewers are rare but it is worthwhile increasing the confidence of interviewers by ensuring that they feel prepared for managing such situations.

Additional resources on risk and safety

- College of Occupational Therapists (September 2003) *Research ethics guidelines*, London: College of Occupational Therapists.
- Social Research Association (2004) 'A code of practice for the safety of social researchers', available from www.the-sra.org.uk

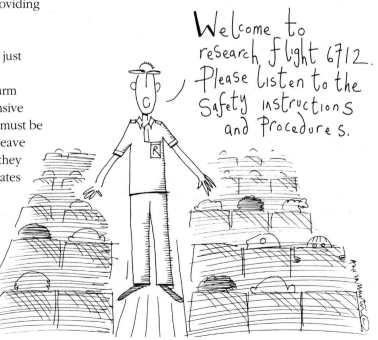

Welcome to research flight 6712. Please listen to the safety instructions and procedures.

6

Involving participants

Involving people with mental health problems in the research process is not the same as involving the actual research participants in the process. The latter represents the epitome of emancipatory research in that it aims to facilitate the active participation and hence potentially the empowerment of those who are traditionally most disempowered by the research process.

Many people consulted for these guidelines spoke from their own experience of being disempowered research 'subjects' and hence of the value they placed on being able to do research differently themselves. This is reflected in many of the suggestions made throughout this chapter. More particularly, some people felt it was important to involve participants in each stage of the research process, for example, identifying research questions, piloting questionnaires, and involving them in the pre-report stage about the analysis and interpretation of the results. Perhaps the issue about which people felt most strongly was that of feedback: too often the passive subject of other people's research and never knowing what came of it, people spoke of the importance of ensuring that research participants receive feedback about the research, including a copy of the report.

Confidentiality

The twin issues of confidentiality and informed consent are those most often addressed in professional guidelines for research as essential protections for research participants, and they figure highly in considerations made by RECs for research approval. Maintaining the confidentiality of research participants is a vital ethical issue and one that signifies our respect to participants.

There are different aspects to confidentiality in research, and it needs to be addressed comprehensively in training and discussion among the research team. There are limits to confidentiality and to anonymity, and it is important that both researchers and participants are clear about these limits.

Data collection

Firstly, the research team need to be clear about what they mean by confidentiality in relation to the data collection. Does it mean that an interviewer will share nothing of the interview they are undertaking with anyone else? This is rarely the case; indeed, for the research to be analysed and reported, it is likely that it will be shared with others in a team. It may mean that the interview will remain anonymous: no names will be attached to any of the information collected, or that names will be held separately and coded in order that participants can be contacted again if required. Confidentiality about who has been involved in the research may be held within a team of researchers, rather than only with the individual carrying out the interview, and this needs to be made quite clear to the participant.

Confidentiality in relation to data collection and retention can usefully be broken down into the following:

- confidentiality and anonymity;
- who will have access to data?
- how will the data be kept? (see the note on the Data Protection Act at the end of this chapter);
- ensuring privacy during research gathering;
- maintaining anonymity: for example, quotations used in the report;

- who will have access to data following publication?

Limits to confidentiality

The limits to confidentiality are the subject of much discussion. It is important to start any interview with a statement about any limits that you may have to maintaining confidentiality, so that the participants can make their own decisions about what they reveal to you. The following potential limits to confidentiality were discussed:

- potential or actual harm to others;
- potential or actual self-harm;
- suicidal intent.

There are legal obligations on all of us to break confidentiality if harm or abuse to children is revealed. Discussion about potential or actual harm to others revealed that most people were in agreement about the need to break confidentiality if they believed there to be a risk of harm to others, or if actual harm currently unknown to others had taken place. (Any intention to break confidentiality should be shared with the participant, unless you believe this will involve risk to yourself.)

Discussions about confidentiality regarding personal disclosure about self-harm or suicidal intent were a great deal lengthier and revealed different views. Several people mentioned spending lengthy training sessions on this subject, despite rarely having to deal with it in practice. It was recognised, however, that it is vital to be prepared for such situations and to have procedures in place for dealing with them, in order that an interviewer can feel confident about managing any potentially difficult situation.

> "In the training confidentiality was the thing that feels hardest. You think about what is the worst case scenario.... "

> "If someone is going to hurt someone or severely hurt themselves I think I would have to talk to them and get them to talk to somebody and then if that's not working I would have to tell them that I would have to breach confidentiality. I have never had to. It would be very rare circumstances."

Professionals in health and social care settings may be clearer about their limits to confidentiality in this respect; they have professional codes of practice with which they need to comply and they have a legal duty of care. However, independent and survivor researchers are not governed by this duty of care, and may have different views about the need to tell a mental health professional about someone's intent to harm themselves if they do not wish you to do so. In this case, it is valid to consider a person's 'best interests'. You may not consider that it is in the person's best interests to tell a mental health professional if they feel that the treatment they will receive as a result will not be helpful to them. However, if someone is suicidal, there may be other routes that you can take or enable them to take, in order that you can leave the situation feeling safe about what has taken place.

If you are concerned about someone harming themself, you could stay with them while they contact a friend or other source of support, or contact someone on their behalf. It is helpful to have a list of local and national support and helplines with you to give to interviewees. This can be something that you leave with them for their own use after you have gone. Finally, it is vital that you have someone to talk to about it afterwards, both for your own support and to talk over other actions you may need to take.

It is important to discuss all of these issues as a team before you start the research: you will need to decide where your shared limits to confidentiality lie in respect of potential self-harm or suicide, and to be clear about the difference between the two. It is also important to set up a support system for interviewers, whereby each one knows whom to contact if they find themselves faced with this kind of dilemma.

Other confidentiality issues

Finally, some additional perspectives on confidentiality arose from certain individual discussions. In forensic services, for example, it was thought important to share certain issues with staff without identifying individuals. Examples given were: illegal drug taking on wards, and instances of bullying or exploitation.

Confidentiality in a broader sense was discussed in the focus group with black participants, where concern was expressed by a couple of people about confidentiality from or within their own communities. This might mean, for example, that

South Asian interviewees would prefer white interviewers in some circumstances, which contradicts assumptions about matching interviewer and interviewee in research. Boundaries of knowledge and confidentiality can be more complex in smaller communities where knowledge might be shared. A similar issue has been raised among small rural communities where research and service provision sometimes need to present themselves in different ways in order to engage and involve people.

"I wrote an article about LGB [lesbian, gay and bisexual] issues among the Asian communities and some Asian people didn't want to talk to me because I was Asian. They felt it was too close to home and I would tell the community. So that may be a consideration."

On a somewhat similar issue, some people talked about the difficulties faced by doing research within their own local mental health communities, and therefore knowing some of the people they were interviewing. This, then, raised another aspect of confidentiality – finding out things about someone in an interview that you would not know about them under usual circumstances, and being able to be clear about the boundaries of these different relationships. This could continue beyond the end of the research project, and needs to be handled with care. Ideally, potential interviewees should be given the choice about whether or not to be interviewed by someone they know, but this may not always be possible.

Suggestions for managing confidentiality

- Discuss it thoroughly in training and preparation for your research and agree your limits to confidentiality as a team (if possible).
- Be clear about what you mean by confidentiality and share your definition, and your limits, with your research participants both in writing and verbally.
- Agree on procedures to follow where a decision needs to be made about breaking confidentiality.
- Whatever you decide, it is essential to share your policy and its limits with participants so that they can make an informed decision.
- Plan for how you might support someone who is intent on harming themselves, for example, help them to contact someone, wait with them while they do so, provide a list of possible helplines and sources of support.

- Check people's preferences about the matching of interviewer with interviewee characteristics such as gender and race or culture; some individuals and some minority ethnic people may not want to be matched on characteristics that might compromise their confidentiality.
- Discuss within the team the implications for confidentiality of interviewing people you know; try to arrange for alternatives if possible.
- With data collection, it is important to think of what happens to the data throughout the research process: collection in privacy, anonymity of data, safe keeping of data, access to data, the presentation of data in reports particularly where qualitative data is concerned, and what happens to data after the research is over.

Informed consent

Informed consent was generally acknowledged as an important issue, again reflecting its status within professional research guidelines. It is a vital means of protection for any of us who may be prospective research participants: knowing what it is that we might be consenting to take part in. It is also a form of protection for researchers: being able to demonstrate that someone has consented to take part in the research. It is generally a condition of RECs that the researchers obtain properly informed consent from participants.

There are two aspects to a basic understanding of informed consent: information and consent. The information about the project needs to be comprehensive and yet accessible in its form and format. Consent can then be freely given or withheld with some confidence. Ideally, information should be given both verbally and in written form, and time should be allowed for people to take in the information if they are being approached about it for the first time. Information about the project needs to include:

- aims of the research;
- information about you and the research team;
- who is funding it;
- what will happen to the research when it is finished;
- feedback to participants;
- confidentiality;
- any risks involved in taking part.

Particular concerns were raised about people held in secure settings feeling able to give their consent freely. However, to some extent these fears were allayed by those carrying out research in forensic settings, where it was found that people were often keen to take part because it meant doing something different or distracting.

> "We did all this work about making sure they knew it was voluntary and we were independent, but when we got there they didn't care and said 'yes I will do it', or 'no I won't' before they even heard about that. It was more about whether they thought they would enjoy the interview or whether research was useful or interesting."

Nevertheless, this is an issue that needs careful consideration, with care taken to ensure that potential participants are aware of the independence of researchers from services and staff, and the value of taking part. It is important to be aware that some patients in secure or inpatient settings may feel that they ought to take part and do not feel able to give their consent freely.

The ways in which informed consent was operated by the survivor researchers consulted for these guidelines varied, with some people placing more emphasis on it than others. In certain contexts, for example, forms were not being used as it was assumed that people did not have to take part if they did not want to. In other circumstances, however, people were more considered about informed consent and felt that participants should be given repeated opportunities to consent to or withdraw from the research, particularly if it was a long-term project. It was also suggested that a distinction be made between withdrawing from the research and discontinuing; in the latter situation, data collected to date might be retained in the research.

> "There should be a right at any stage to withdraw – at any stage including at the transcript stage."

Some people spent considerable time with people on wards or in other residential settings, in order to ensure that prospective participants would get to know them and perhaps come to trust in the research they were carrying out. This meant more opportunities to explain what it was about and to ensure that people were aware of what they were consenting to. Similarly some people talked of presenting the research in a group first, and then approaching people individually for consent.

To some extent, these differences will depend on whether a project is officially termed 'research' or not; if it is an audit or monitoring exercise, it will not necessarily need to comply with the requirements of an REC on procedures for obtaining informed consent. However, good practice would suggest that people get as full information as possible about any project they may be approached to take part in.

Suggestions for informed consent

- Think about the *information* as well as the *consent* in informed consent: give people clear and accessible written and verbal information about your project.
- Check that people understand what it is that they are consenting to take part in.
- Think about the context in which your participants are to be approached: are they held in a secure setting or environment in which their freely given consent might be compromised? If so, try spending time with people to engage their interest in the project in advance of approaching them individually.
- In a long-term project, give participants the opportunity to consent or withdraw at key points in the project.

Support for participants

This was one of the key issues for survivor researchers consulted for these guidelines. Most people felt strongly about the need to have a range of things in place to ensure that participants are not caused undue harm by research, and are given ample opportunity to withdraw at any stage. Nevertheless, several people expressed the view that participants may not object to being distressed by an interview, and it should not be assumed that this should be avoided at all costs:

> "Becoming distressed is not the same as harm."

> " … because with some people it can be the first time that anyone has asked them and they can be really distressed and you can ask if they want to stop the interview and they'll say no. Although it can be uncomfortable seeing people distressed, we have to recognise that by giving them a voice we may be serving another function."

For many people, it was their own experience at the receiving end of other people's research that motivated them to think about the importance of supporting research participants. In my experience of working with service users and survivors in many different projects, people are always careful to think and reflect about this issue and its implications.

A key issue is the need to gauge whether or not a potential participant is too vulnerable to take part in the first place. There may be some indications that it is not appropriate to interview someone, for example, if a person is actively distressed or is not able to understand fully the nature of what is taking place. Although the latter should become clear when attempting to obtain informed consent prior to an interview, it is possible that it may not. (An example was given of an interviewee continuing to mistake the interviewer for a service provider some time into the interview; in this case, the interview was cut short and not used in the research.) If someone is actively distressed at the time of the interview, it may be possible to suggest an alternative time and date for interview; if so, it is suggested that you put this in writing or contact them again later.

Some people talked of the importance of not leaving participants feeling worse after an interview than they felt beforehand: for example, taking time at the end of the interview to talk informally or to have a cup of tea, so that the ending is not abrupt. Most people recommended preparing a list of contacts to take into all interviews, in order to provide participants with possible local resources or helplines that they could contact afterwards. Occasionally, researchers had been asked by a participant directly for advice or information, which conflicted with their role as researcher or interviewer. A list of local resources and helplines, including advocacy services, is a simple way to help in this situation and avoid being drawn into helping someone with an individual problem.

The context and subject of the research has some bearing on the need for support. If you are undertaking research with people in hospital or in a vulnerable situation, then the need to have some forms of support available will be greater. Similarly, if you know your subject to be a sensitive one and to be a possible cause of distress, then it is all the more important to think of ways of managing this. However, it is always a possibility that participants will wish to talk about their personal story and become distressed while doing so.

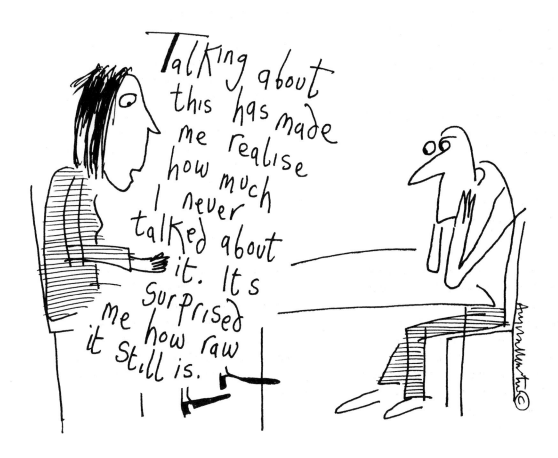

Suggestions for supporting participants

- Send advance information about the project and your intended visit or invitation to interview (by post, leaflet or meeting, depending on the context). Carry some form of ID and a 'phone number for interviewees to check your identity if required. Give participants a list of contact numbers for relevant resources or helplines, and consider exploring these with someone who is distressed or suicidal.
- Reassure participants that they do not need to answer a question(s) if they do not wish to.
- Be prepared to take a break from interviewing if the participant becomes upset or distressed.
- Take time at the end of the interview to talk informally, and perhaps have a cup of tea with them.
- If the participant is very distressed, check if they would like you to contact someone for them.
- Think about options for follow-up after an interview; several people said that they have offered this occasionally – either a follow-up visit or a 'phone call to check and debrief a little while after the interview.
- However, be careful to maintain your boundaries or some sense of your own role in the interaction: you are a researcher (or interviewer), not a carer or counsellor in this situation.

Payment to participants

It was generally agreed that participants should be offered some incentives for taking part in research: payment for expenses and for time, and feedback about the research findings. Payment for expenses (such as travel, care and subsistence costs) was agreed to be essential. There was a little more discussion about payment as recognition for people's time and experience.

It has become more common for people to be paid for taking part in research in recent years. Most people spoke of paying people within the range of £10-£20 (in 2003) for an individual or group interview, and sometimes more if expert advice was being acknowledged. There were exceptions to this, where people in secure institutions were either not paid at all or were paid less than the average. In one instance, this was due to rules forbidding payment:

"Their view is that they'll only turn up for the money but you still get the information, but most don't do it for that reason but because they want to tell you what's happening. You only get a few extra for the money. It is important to value people. We can do it with community services and with acute but there must be a way of doing it in forensic. In [X] I bought a video game for the ward."

In another, it was due to the views of the service user researcher, who felt that too much money would influence people unduly:

"We were able to give them £5 for the interview. In the other ones we gave £10 but those in the secure hospital get so little money that G thought they might just do it for the money, then talk for 5 minutes and then go."

As with the discussion about paying researchers and interviewers, the need for some degree of flexibility was acknowledged. Payment was not always possible, for example, for those engaged in higher education or in small projects or groups with few resources. In these situations, people advocated some creativity on the part of researchers in thinking about what could be offered to participants. Examples given were: newsletters or other publications, a meal or refreshments, a copy of the research report or the opportunity to take part in a conference, training or other activity.

While some measure of flexibility was acknowledged to be necessary, it was emphasised that funded projects, or projects seeking funding, should include payments to participants in their budget. Choice should be given to participants as to how this payment can best be made; for example, it may be easier for some people to receive payment by tokens or vouchers in place of cash.

Note: the 1998 Data Protection Act

The requirements of the 1998 Data Protection Act must be adhered to where appropriate. The Act gives individuals rights regarding the personal data held about them by organisations and gives organisations responsibilities regarding the protection and use of that data. The Data Protection Act contains eight Principles. These state that all data must be:

- processed fairly and lawfully;
- obtained and used only for specified and lawful purposes;
- adequate, relevant and not excessive;
- accurate and, where necessary, kept up to date;
- kept for no longer than necessary;
- processed in accordance with the individuals' rights (as defined);
- kept secure;
- transferred only to countries that offer adequate data protection.

There are exemptions relating to the use of data for research purposes and it is advisable to obtain advice if you are in any doubt. For example, if research data are completely anonymised such that it is not possible to identify the individuals concerned, then the research may be exempt from the Act. Advice may be obtained from www.hmso.gov.uk/acts/acts1998/19980029.htm or from your local university, NHS trust or local authority, each of which will have a Data Protection Officer.

7

Analysis and feedback

Analysis and interpretation

Having collected the data or information from participants, there is a question about how we, as researchers, treat or deal with that data in an ethical way. The respect that we held for participants needs to be followed through by respecting the information they shared with us. Participants in the black focus group were particularly concerned about how researchers analyse and interpret their findings with respect for black communities. They referred to the several research studies which have investigated mental illness in minority ethnic communities and interpreted it differently to how black communities or black researchers might interpret it.

In the guidelines for ethical mental health research involving issues of race, ethnicity and culture (Patel, 1999), the author suggests that researchers be encouraged to be "explicit about their rationale and methods of data analysis so that the research is more open to scrutiny for potential bias. Such bias may otherwise pass unnoticed and result in the outcome of the research being unquestioned and perhaps inappropriately applied". Early on in the present guidelines, we have accepted that all researchers do have some degree of bias, or a perspective that influences the research they undertake. Nevertheless, the approach suggested here does give readers the opportunity to understand the perspective taken by researchers and is, I would argue, particularly important in relation to qualitative research where the analysis is sometimes not made explicit (although it can be[2]).

Referring back to the vital issue of confidentiality (see Chapter 6), this is the time when it is

important to remember that direct quotations may have the power to identify individuals in your research report. If you think that this is a possibility, then it is important to check back with the individual(s) concerned. It may be that they do not object to the possibility of identification at this stage; however, if they do object or if it is not possible to check back with them and confidentiality was guaranteed, then the quotation must be discarded.

There are a number of measures that can be taken to demonstrate how you have approached the analysis of your data and arrived at your conclusions:

- Be open about your theoretical approach and any prior views you held about the topic (see Chapter 2, Underlying principles).
- Give a clear account of the process you adopted to analyse your data: show how you arrived at your themes or codes, and use examples to illustrate.
- If appropriate, work as a team and check your coding and interpretations with each other.
- Take your analysis back to the research participants and incorporate their comments into the final discussion.
- If you use a number of different research methods (for example, interviews and questionnaires) you can 'triangulate' the data and see how the findings from different approaches compare or complement each other.

Feedback to participants

Feedback to participants was one of the issues that gave rise to particularly strong feelings on the part of people interviewed for these guidelines. Many had been involved in research as participants

---

[2] See, for example, the session on analysis in Nicholls et al (1999).

themselves and felt quite angry that they had never received either proper feedback about the research findings or a copy of the final report. They therefore highlighted this as an important principle for survivor research, and one that signifies respect to our participants.

> "It's important because in my experience you never used to get any feedback and it really gets to you and so you never wanted to take part any more … you have a duty to share the results back."

For some people, feedback meant sending participants a copy of the final research report, whereas for others it meant ensuring accessible feedback in a shorter format. This may depend on resources as well as on the need for accessibility. Research findings may be written in a format suitable for an academic audience or for policy makers and may need to be written up in a more accessible format for feeding back to participants. In some cases, however, the same report may be given to all stakeholders in the research. Either way, there were strong feelings among those consulted for these guidelines that feedback to participants should be part of the deal in carrying out research.

> "Research shouldn't be done if there's no intention to get back to the participants."

Feedback to participants is held to be particularly important by the Strategies for Living project. They have encouraged researchers to involve participants in consultations about the findings, and to check back with people that they are happy with the way in which they have been represented in the report. An example was given of the Somerset Spirituality project, in which a consultation day was held for participants to see and to hear about the findings in progress (research reported in Somerset Spirituality Project Research Team and Nicholls, 2002).

Suggestions for feedback:

- If resources allow, involve participants at a half-way stage in the analysis, giving them the opportunity to comment on your analysis and interpretation.
- Ensure that your research participants receive accessible feedback about the research findings and a copy of the full report if they want one.
- Consider providing participants with information about other publications that arise from the research.

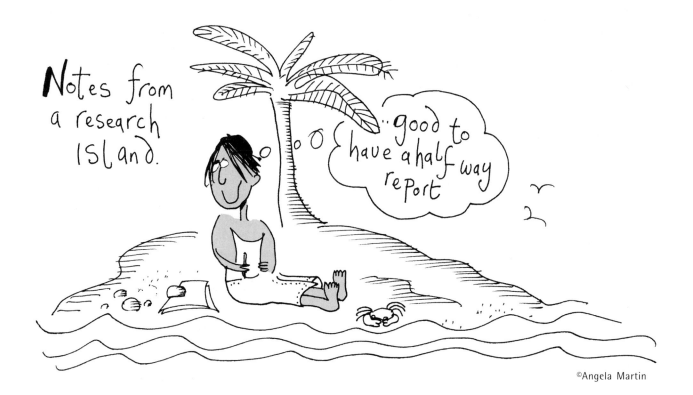

©Angela Martin

8

Dissemination and implementation

Dissemination

Dissemination is the outward-looking presentation of research findings: how you tell other people, whether or not they were involved in the research, what you found out through the research and why or how it is important. As with feedback to participants, dissemination gave rise to strong feelings of principle on the part of those consulted for these guidelines. It is regarded by many as a *duty* to disseminate the findings of research, to make them publicly available particularly to the relevant stakeholders. However, occasions were reported where survivors have been in difficulties at the time of dissemination and needed to find other ways or other people to assist with writing up and disseminating the findings.

It is useful to consider *written* dissemination in relation to different perspectives, audiences or stakeholders:

- report of the findings to funders and others involved in the research project;
- articles in relevant practice journals to influence policy makers and practitioners;
- articles in academic journals;
- accessible report or summary of findings to reach wider audience of local stakeholders, service users and carers who may be interested in or affected by the research findings;
- articles or mentions in mental health journals and newsletters that reach mental health service users and survivors;
- Internet publication.

Examples of effective accessible dissemination include: summaries of Strategies for Living research projects (see the Mental Health Foundation website: www.mentalhealth.org.uk); and the Joseph Rowntree Foundation Findings series (www.jrf.org.uk).

Some of the most accessible reports are not formally published or are published locally: for example, local projects and service evaluations. Most of the full reports of the projects supported by the Strategies for Living programme have been published locally, with summary documents held on the website; for example:

- Walsh, J. and Boyle, J. (2003) 'Improving acute psychiatric hospital services according to inpatient experiences' [copies of the full report likely to be available from the Derriaghy Centre in Northern Ireland].
- Bodman, R. et al (2003) *Life's labours lost: A study of the experiences of people who have lost their occupation following mental health problems* [copies available from the UFM Project at Bristol Mind, the Mental Health Foundation's website or the Bristol Mind website: www.bristolmind.org.uk].

The Service User Research Enterprise at the Institute of Psychiatry has experience of dissemination in academic journals, as well as of making research results available to service users through other routes. For example, their review of consumers' perspectives of ECT was published as an article in the *British Medical Journal* (Rose et al, 2003), and in the Mind magazine *Openmind* (Fleischmann et al, 2003) and the report was used to influence the guidelines on ECT produced by NICE (the National Institute for Clinical Excellence).

When considering accessibility it is important to look at the relevant audiences or stakeholders that you need to reach; for example, if you translated research materials into a language other than English, it is important to do the same with your research findings in order that those same people can have access to the research results.

Another consideration concerns the best methods of reaching different minority groups affected by your research. It may be appropriate to seek to disseminate via magazines or journals aimed at specific black or minority ethnic communities, or lesbian and gay communities, for example. Some communities may be better reached through different routes; for example, radio programmes might be a more effective route for reaching some minority communities, the Internet for others. You need to make sure that you know your own audiences or find out about them in order that you can choose the most appropriate routes for dissemination.

Oral dissemination can often reach people that written dissemination does not. It is all too easy to order a report and place it on a shelf unread, but a good oral presentation at a conference can be more effective in some instances. Equally, conferences may only attract people who are already interested in your research. Organising a local event for stakeholders and members of the public interested in the subject of your research may be a more effective means of bringing about change. Another potential route is to take findings in person to the people who might be able to implement them: to arrange meetings with local professionals, service managers or policy makers who could take notice of your research findings and act on them.

Some options for dissemination

- presentation at a relevant conference or seminar;
- organising your own conference to launch the research findings;
- organising a local event for all stakeholders with an interest in your subject;
- meeting with local or national policy makers or service managers;
- radio, video or television media.

Implementation of research

"What is the point of doing research if it's not implementable?"

Remembering Chapter 2 (Underlying principles), the research for these guidelines found that survivor researchers feel strongly that research should have a *commitment to change*. The ethical implementation of research in this context implies being true to the findings and bringing about change that service users want. Implementation of research results is a challenge for many researchers, both academic and otherwise; many would like to see their research results implemented, but few researchers will be in a position to do so themselves because of the limitations of their role.

Time and resources are needed to implement research effectively, but there may be ways in which it can be built in from the start. Action research and service evaluations both assume a role for the implementation of findings – a complete research cycle, in effect. For example, it is one of the criteria for the UFM projects that they engage local services in a commitment to change in response to the findings: one of their aims is "*to make positive changes in mental health services and generate creative alternatives to existing services*" (italics for emphasis).

Between May 2001 and May 2002 the UFM Project based at Bristol Mind conducted research into service users' experiences of being inpatients. This research was published in a report: 'User focused study of inpatient services in three Bristol hospitals' (Bristol Mind UFM Project, 2004). The findings in this report and the recommendations for change were presented to service users and providers. The report also led to the formation of an implementation group that aims to ensure that the recommendations in the report are acted on.

The work of ARW in forensic mental health services has led to practical changes in conditions for people in forensic services, such as an extra occupational therapist and lighting in a courtyard. More fundamentally perhaps, ARW believe that they have brought about a change in attitudes among the staff towards the users of their services.

One of the suggestions made by Strategies for Living researchers was to ask for feedback from policy makers or managers to whom the research has been disseminated: invite a dialogue about how the findings might be acted on. An example is given in the following box of the Somerset Spirituality Project, a project in which the research findings were implemented in a number of different ways. This was largely due to local commitment to the project on behalf of the Trust which provided some of the funding, but also to the commitment of all those involved to the issues raised by the research.

Implementation of research: the Somerset Spirituality Project

1. The research

This research was initiated by a group of people coming together who shared a common interest in religious and spiritual needs and resources and a shared experience of using mental health services in Somerset. Training and support was provided by Vicky Nicholls (and, in the first year, Alison Faulkner) from the Mental Health Foundation Strategies for Living project. Interviews took place with 27 people in Somerset; these were all taped and 25 transcribed for the purposes of analysis (two were withdrawn by participants). The project was funded jointly by the local Trust and the Mental Health Foundation. The questions addressed by the research were as follows:

- How do service users/survivors experience and manage their mental health problems and their religious and spiritual needs?
- What help or hindrance have they had for this from the mental health services of Somerset?
- What help or hindrance have they had from local religious and spiritual groups and individuals?
- How important has acceptance been for them in this?

2. Recommendations

The research was published by the Mental Health Foundation in the report *Taken seriously: The Somerset Spirituality Project* (Somerset Spirituality Project Research Team and Nicholls, 2002). A number of recommendations were made, of which the following are just a few:

To people working in mental health services:
- Help service users to identify their important values, beliefs and practices, including what helps them cope with and understand their mental health problems spiritually and religiously.
- Provide access to religious and spiritual resources; for example chaplaincy services, safe opportunities to discuss these issues, a safe space or place where people can pray, meditate, practise their faith.

To managers and planners:
- Include awareness training of beliefs and practices of different faiths and spiritual traditions in the training of all mental health professionals.
- Ensure staff are aware of relevant local resources for service users with particular religious or spiritual needs, including people within mental health services and knowledgeable and sensitive contacts in faith communities.

To people in faith communities:
- Offer practical help and support; these are often needed and appreciated.
- Respect, value and try to understand the beliefs of others if they are different from your own.
- Include rather than exclude service users; encourage rather than discourage.

To ministers and other religious/spiritual leaders:
- Offer opportunities for non-judgemental listening and talking through issues.
- Pray with service users, if invited or permission given.

3. Implementation of the research

- The local Trust has made a commitment to introduce safe quiet spaces into all acute services.
- Local and national conferences took place.
- Several spirituality groups have been set up, for example in Taunton and Glastonbury. These are cross-sector groups with service users, social workers, chaplains and carers involved.
- A two-day event was organised in Yeovil for people with shared interests to spend time together.
- A special edition of the *Journal of Mental Health, Religion and Culture* has been published on the Somerset Project (vol 7, no 1, March 2004).
- Members of the group continue to speak at conferences and workshops.
- A post, established within the Mental Health Foundation focusing on mental health and spirituality, has been part-funded by the National Institute for Mental Health (England).

9

Research Ethics Committees

The government's *Research Governance Framework* (DH, 2001) states that the dignity, rights, safety and well-being of participants must be the primary consideration in any research study. Research which takes place within the NHS has to be approved by an NHS REC, but there is currently no clear system of ethical review for social care research. The Department of Health has recently (May 2004) produced an implementation plan for research governance in social care research (DH, 2004).

RECs have a number of professional members and usually one lay member and they meet on a regular basis to consider research proposals. They have fixed submission dates, and can ask researchers to resubmit to a future meeting with changes to their proposal. It is best to be prepared for possible delays at this stage. To find out meeting dates, it is possible to contact your Trust HQ and ask for the Committee administrator.

The chief concerns of ethics committees are that participants should not be harmed by the research (a principle often called 'non-maleficence'), that the research is for the common good ('beneficence'), and that confidentiality be maintained and fully informed consent obtained. This *can* result in overly protective or paternalistic committees unwilling to consider research that may upset people (see the note on protection from harm at the end of Chapter 2). In the consultation for developing research ethics for social care, it was argued that the current system of RECs was designed to protect vulnerable people, rather than to hear their voices and support a greater role for service users in research. RECs are also concerned with the safety of researchers, so your proposal should include a description of any arrangements

for ensuring your own and other researchers' safety in order to avoid possible delay.

In reality, RECs vary quite considerably because they have different members with different views and strictly speaking share no common guidelines. Hence, in some areas, there may be members who are familiar with mental health research, the involvement of service users or consumers in research and with qualitative research – and in others there may not.

One of the people consulted for these guidelines had experience of gaining approval for a research project from a REC, and emphasised the importance of covering every possible eventuality from the point of view of potential harm or risk.

> "We were very thorough about what were the risks, everything from upset interviewees, upset researchers, violence, confidentiality, risk of G being isolated by other patients. We put down all the possible risks and what steps we had taken to deal with it."

It also helped that they had letters of support from people with academic research experience, and that they had received help from academic researchers in filling in the relevant forms. In the end,

> "I was pleased that the committee took us seriously, had considered the relevant ethical issues, and did not patronise us at all. They were also very positive about user-led research, calling it 'innovative' and wishing us luck with the project."

However, these preparations may not always work. Sadly, a couple of the Strategies for Living projects had to be abandoned early on because they did not receive ethical approval. Burke (2002) wrote of his experience of a REC:

> The end result seems to have turned a valuable, well overdue and relatively simple project into a convoluted and unnecessarily complicated piece of research.

The respondents to our questionnaire felt that the process of application should be simplified and made more 'user-friendly'. They also felt that full feedback should be given to applicants and that there should be a complaints procedure and/or appeals procedure in place for those not satisfied with decisions. Issues proposed that were not on the original list were: that committees should give quick decisions, and that they should become "more appropriate to different types of research". This last is important since the application forms assume a particular research approach: the randomised controlled trial will fit in to the questions much more easily than a qualitative study.

The Department of Health consultation with service users that took place for the development of ethical guidelines for social care research came up with a number of further recommendations, including:

- a user-led reference group for COREC;
- a register of social care ethical researchers managed by a user-led organisation;
- peer review of research proposals by service users;
- if users are to be involved on RECs or other committees, then they need training and support to make the most of their roles.

The role of a Research Ethics Committee

RECs are the committees convened to provide the independent advice to participants, researchers, funders, sponsors, employers, care organisations and professionals on the extent to which proposals for research studies comply with recognised ethical standards.

The purpose of a REC in reviewing the proposed study is to protect the dignity, rights, safety and well-being of all actual or potential research participants. It shares this role and responsibility with others, as described in the *Research Governance Framework for Health and Social Care* (from the COREC website: www.corec.org.uk/public/about/about.htm)

References

Barnes, C. and Mercer, G. (eds) (1997) *Doing disability research*, Leeds: Disability Press.

Beresford, P. and Wallcraft, J. (1997) 'Psychiatric system survivors and emancipatory research: issues, overlaps and differences', in C. Barnes and G. Mercer (eds) *Doing disability research*, Leeds: Disability Press.

Bristol Mind UFM Project (2004) 'User focused study of inpatient services in three Bristol hospitals' (www.bristolmind.org.uk).

Burke, M. (2002) 'A service user/researcher's experience with an Ethics Committee', *Consumers in NHS Support Unit Areas*, Spring, Eastleigh: INVOLVE.

Danley, K. and Ellison, M.L. (1999) *Handbook for participatory researchers*, Boston: Center for Psychiatric Rehabilitation.

DH (Department of Health) (2001) *Research Governance Framework for Health and Social Care*, London: DH.

DH (2004) *Research Governance Framework for Health and Social Care: Implementation Plan for Social Care*, London: DH

Faulkner, A. and Layzell, S. (2000) *Strategies for living: A report of user-led research into people's strategies for living with mental distress*, London: Mental Health Foundation.

Fleischmann, P., Rose, D. and Wykes T. (2003) 'Life saver or memory eraser?', *Openmind*, no 122, July/August, pp 12-13.

Nicholls, V., Faulkner, A. and Blazdell, J. (1999) *The DIY guide to survivor research*, London: Mental Health Foundation.

Patel, N. (1999) *Getting the evidence: Guidelines for ethical mental health research involving issues of 'race', ethnicity and culture*, London: Mind/Trans-Cultural Psychiatry Society.

Rose, D. (2001) *Users' voices: The perspectives of mental health service users on community and hospital care*, London: Sainsbury Centre for Mental Health.

Rose, D., Fleischmann, P., Wykes, T., Leese, M. and Bindman, J. (2003) 'Patients' perspectives on electroconvulsive therapy: systematic review', *British Medical Journal*, 21 June, vol 326, no 7403, p 1363.

Somerset Spirituality Project Research Team and Nicholls, V. (2002) *Taken seriously: The Somerset Spirituality Project*, London: Mental Health Foundation.

UFM Network (2003) *Doing it for real: A guide to setting up and undertaking a User Focused Monitoring project*, London: Sainsbury Centre for Mental Health (www.scmh.org.uk).

Further reading and contact details for organisations mentioned in the text

Barnes, C. and Mercer, G. (eds) (1997) *Doing disability research*, Leeds: Disability Press.

Beresford, P. (2002) 'User involvement in research and evaluation: liberation or regulation?', *Social Policy and Society*, vol 1, no 2, pp 95-105.

Beresford, P. and Evans, C. (1999) 'Research note: research and empowerment', *British Journal of Social Work*, vol 29, pp 671-7.

Beresford, P. and Wallcraft, J. (1997) 'Psychiatric system survivors and emancipatory research: issues, overlaps and differences', in C. Barnes and G. Mercer (eds) *Doing disability research*, Leeds: Disability Press.

Bodman, R., Davies, R., Frankel, N., Minton, L., Mitchell, L., Pacé, C., Sayers, R., Tibbs, N., Tovey, Z. and Unger, E. (2003) *Life's labours lost: A study of the experiences of people who have lost their occupation following mental health problems*, Bristol: UFM Project, Bristol Mind (www.bristolmind.org.uk or www.mentalhealth.org.uk).

Boote, J., Telford, R. and Cooper, C. (2002) 'Consumer involvement in health research: a review and research agenda', *Health Policy*, vol 61, pp 213-36.

Carrick, R., Mitchell, A. and Lloyd, K. (2001) 'User involvement in research: power and compromise', *Journal of Community & Applied Social Psychology*, vol 11, pp 217-25.

Clark, C.C., Scott, E.A., Boydell, K.M. and Goering, R. (1999) 'Effects of client interviewers on client-reported satisfaction with mental health services', *Psychiatric Services*, vol 50, no 7, pp 961-3.

College of Occupational Therapists (September 2003) *Research ethics guidelines*.

Crawford, M.J., Rutter, D., Manley, C., Bhui K., Weaver, T., Fulop, N. and Tyre, P. (2001) *User involvement in the planning and delivery of mental health services*, report to London Region NHSE, London: National Health Service Executive.

Davies, A. and Braithwaite, T. (2001) 'In our own hands: a research network for service users/survivors aims to be a powerful forum for change', *Mental Health Care*, vol 4, no 12.

Denscombe, M. (1998) *The good research guide for small-scale research projects*, Buckingham: Open University Press.

DH (Department of Health) (2001) *Research Governance Framework for Health and Social Care*, London: DH.

Faulkner, A. (1997) *Knowing our own minds*, London: Mental Health Foundation.

Faulkner, A. (in press) *Capturing the experiences of those involved in the TRUE Project: A story of colliding worlds*, Eastleigh: INVOLVE (www.invo.org.uk).

Faulkner, A. and Layzell, S. (2000) *Strategies for living: A report of user-led research into people's strategies for living with mental distress*, London: Mental Health Foundation.

Faulkner, A. and Morris, B. (2003) *Expert paper: User involvement in forensic mental health research and development*, National Programme on Forensic Mental Health Research and Development, Liverpool.

Faulkner, A. and Thomas, P. (2002) 'User-led research and evidence based medicine', *British Journal of Psychiatry*, vol 180, pp 1-3.

Hanley, B., Bradburn, J., Barnes, M., Evans, C., Goodare, H., Kelson, M., Kent, A., Oliver, S., Thomas, S. and Wallcraft, J. (2003) *Involving the public in NHS, public health and social care research: Briefing notes for researchers* (2nd edn), Eastleigh: INVOLVE.

INVOLVE (2003) 'A guide to paying members of the public who are actively involved in research' (www.invo.org.uk).

Lindow, V. (2002) 'Being ethical, having influence', *Openmind*, no 116, pp 18-19.

Lindow, V., Lockey, R., Sitzia, J., Gillingham, T., Millyard, J., Miller, C., Ahmed, S., Beales, A., Bennett, C., Parfoot, S., Sigrist, G. and Sigrist, J. (2001) 'Survival research', in C. Newnes, G. Holmes and C. Dunn (eds) *This is madness too*, Ross-on-Wye: PCCS Books, pp 135-46.

Lockey, R. et al (2004) *Training for service user involvement in health and social care research: A study of training provision and participants' experiences (the TRUE Project)*, Worthing: Worthing and Southlands Hospitals NHS Trust.

Martyn, D. in collaboration with 48 people with a schizophrenia diagnosis (2001) *The experiences and views of self-management of people with a schizophrenia diagnosis*, London: Rethink.

Mental Health Foundation (2003) *A fair day's pay: A guide to benefits, service user involvement and payments*, London: Mental Health Foundation (www.mentalhealth.org.uk).

Nicholls, V. (2001) *Doing research ourselves*, London: Mental Health Foundation.

Nicholls, V. et al (1999) *The DIY guide to survivor research*, London: Mental Health Foundation.

Nicholls V. et al (2003) *Surviving user-led research: Reflections on supporting user-led research projects*, London: Mental Health Foundation.

Oliver, M. (1992) 'Changing the social relationship of research production?', *Disability, Handicap and Society*, vol 7, no 2, pp 101-14.

Openmind no 116, July/August 2002, *Full speed ahead? The state of user research* (whole issue), London: Mind Publications.

Polowycz, D. et al (1993) 'Comparison of patient and staff surveys of consumer satisfaction', *Hospital and Community Psychiatry*, vol 44, no 6, pp 589-691.

Ramon, S. (2000) 'Participative mental health research: users and professional researchers working together', *Mental Health Care*, vol 3, no 7, pp 224-8.

Rose, D. (1996) *Living in the community*, London: Sainsbury Centre for Mental Health.

Rose, D. (2001) *Users' voices: The perspectives of mental health service users on community and hospital care*, London: Sainsbury Centre for Mental Health.

Rose, D. (2003) 'Collaborative research between users and professionals: peaks and pitfalls', *Psychiatric Bulletin*, vol 27, pp 404-6.

Rose, D. et al and the KCW Mental Health Monitoring Users' Group (1998) *In our experience: User Focused Monitoring of mental health services in Kensington & Chelsea and Westminster Health Authority*, London: Sainsbury Centre for Mental Health.

Royle, J. et al (2001) *Getting involved in research: A guide for consumers*, Eastleigh: Consumers in NHS Research Support Unit, available from INVOLVE.

Simpson, E. and House, A.O. (2002) 'Involving users in the delivery and evaluation of mental health services: systematic review', *British Medical Journal*, 30 November, vol 325, p 1265.

Social Research Association (2004) 'A code of practice for the safety of social researchers', available from www.the-sra.org.uk

Somerset Spirituality Project Research Team and Nicholls, V. (2002) *Taken seriously: The Somerset Spirituality Project*, London: Mental Health Foundation.

Telford, R. et al (2002) 'Consumer involvement in health research: fact or fiction?', *British Journal of Clinical Governance*, vol 7, no 2, pp 92-103.

Thornicroft, G. et al (2002) 'What are the research priorities of mental health service users?', *Journal of Mental Health*, vol 11, no 1, pp 1-5.

Townend, M. and Braithwaite, T. (2002) 'Mental health research – the value of user involvement', *Journal of Mental Health*, vol 11, no 2, pp 117-19.

Trivedi, P. and Wykes, T. (2002) 'From passive subjects to equal partners', *British Journal of Psychiatry*, vol 181, pp 468-72.

UFM Network (2003) *Doing it for real: A guide to setting up and undertaking a User Focused Monitoring project*, London: Sainsbury Centre for Mental Health (www.scmh.org.uk).

Walsh, J. and Boyle, J. (2003) 'Improving acute psychiatric hospital services according to inpatient experiences' (www.mentalhealth.org.uk).

Contact details for organisations mentioned in the text

Advocacy Really Works (ARW)
27, Ladyfields
Loughton
Essex
IG10 3RP
Tel 020 8502 3132
e-mail: advocacy@reallyworks.fsnet.co.uk

Bristol Mind
PO Box 1174
Bristol
BS99 2PQ
Tel 0117 373 0336
www.bristolmind.org.uk

INVOLVE
Wessex House
Upper Market Street
Eastleigh
Hampshire
SO50 9FD
Tel 023 8065 1088
www.invo.org.uk

Joseph Rowntree Foundation
The Homestead
40 Water End
York
YO30 6WP
Tel 01904 629241
www.jrf.org.uk

Mental Health Foundation
7th Floor
83 Victoria Street
London
SW1H 0HN
Tel 020 7802 0300
www.mentalhealth.org.uk

Sainsbury Centre for Mental Health
134-138 Borough High Street
London
SE1 1LB
Tel 020 7403 8790
www.scmh.org.uk

Service User Research Enterprise
PO34
Health Services Research Department
Institute of Psychiatry
De Crespigny Park
Denmark Hill
London
SE5 8AF
Tel 020 7848 5104

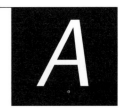

Appendix A:
The research

The research project

This one-year project was funded by the Joseph Rowntree Foundation and was proposed originally by Viv Lindow (Survivor Researcher). The project aimed to develop an accessible manual for ethical practice for researchers, trainers in research skills and interviewers working from the perspective of mental health service users and survivors.

In recent years, there has been a considerable increase in both local and national user/survivor research projects and initiatives. Government policy has supported this through the *Research Governance Framework* (DH, 2001), which encourages consumer involvement in all stages of the research process. In addition, or as a result, many research funders are increasingly calling for academic research to involve consumers as a condition of funding.

There is evidence of much local activity in the form of individual projects, as well as larger initiatives to support the development of user/survivor research. There is a distinction to be made between survivor-controlled research and 'user involvement in research', but many of the ethical issues will be very similar. While some materials have been developed to support these initiatives (by, for example, the Mental Health Foundation and the Sainsbury Centre for Mental Health UFM Network), a 'code of practice' has not emerged. This was considered particularly important in order to ensure and encourage the development of good practice.

Aims

- To develop a code of practice and accompanying guidance, for survivor researchers and interviewers and for trainers.

- In the process of developing this, to consult widely with survivor researchers and interviewers nationwide, in order to ensure a broad input to the code of practice.

Methods

The project engaged the following methods in order to ensure that the manual would draw on sources of expertise in this area:

- a literature review to discover: existing professional research codes of practice, survivor researcher projects, and research experience of other discriminated-against groups such as black, gay and lesbian, disabled and feminist researchers;
- a series of individual interviews and focus groups around the UK;
- a questionnaire to a sample of survivor researchers.

In addition, a reference group of survivor researchers was convened from people with differing perspectives to guide the consultation process. This combination of methods was chosen in order that the manual would not attempt to reinvent the wheel, but would incorporate elements of the existing research codes of practice of professional groups and the experience of researchers working in this and related fields.

It was also thought that focus groups (or group interviews) would facilitate a number of people in one location or involved in one project to spark off experiences and ideas from each other. Individual interviews, on the other hand, would enable the expertise of experienced survivor researchers to be included in the manual.

It was hoped that the nationwide nature of the project and its emphasis on consultation would assist with ownership of the code of practice, and alert survivor researchers to the future publication of the manual.

Sample achieved

a) Focus groups

The following focus groups were carried out:

Focus group	Location	Comments
1. Mental Health Foundation (MHF) Strategies for Living core support team	London	Focus group in London; some members of team from other parts of the UK
2. Making Waves	Nottingham	UFM group based in Nottingham
3. Bristol Mind UFM	Bristol, South West	UFM team based at Bristol Mind
4. MHF Strategies for Living Scotland and Northern Ireland team	Glasgow, Scotland	Mixed team of researchers and advisory group members from Strategies for Living projects in Scotland and Northern Ireland
5. Black focus group	London	Members of the group came from different projects, backgrounds and experiences
6. TRUE Project (Training in Research skills for service Users: project Evaluation)	Worthing, Sussex	All team members had been involved in a research project together, funded by INVOLVE

b) Individual interviews

Interview	Location	Comments
1. Peter Beresford	London	Professor at Brunel University, and Chair of Shaping Our Lives
2. David Armes	London	PhD Student
3. Nutan Kotecha	London	Sainsbury Centre: UFM Coordinator
4. Nasa Begum	London	Policy Officer, Mind
5. Roberta Wetherell	Essex	Director of ARW (Advocacy Really Works); forensic services experience
6. Rachel Waters	Cardiff, South Wales	Strategies for Living support worker for Wales
7. Mick Burke	Essex	Interview pending due to illness

c) Questionnaire respondents

The 15 questionnaire respondents described themselves as follows, the majority being user/survivor researchers (13):

Researcher	13	
Interviewer	11	
Trainer	9	
User/survivor	15	
Academic	3	
Mental health worker/professional	6	
Other (please state)	Human being	1
	Committee member	1

The 11 people who gave their addresses came from the following parts of the UK:

London (5)
Hampshire
Worcestershire
South Wales (2)
Hertfordshire
Bristol

The sample was biased towards London and the South of England, which is in part due to the concentration of survivor researchers in these regions, particularly those from black and minority ethnic communities.

Ethnicity

The ethnic profile of the sample was as follows. Two of the six individual interviewees were South Asian women. Two of the four members of the black focus group were South Asian (one man and one woman), the other two were Black African Caribbean women, and the co-facilitator was an Asian woman. There was one Asian male participant in the TRUE Project focus group.

Design of research schedules

The *Handbook for participatory action researchers* (Danley and Ellison, 1999) is fascinating, and well worth a read. It is based on a fairly large-scale project carried out as participatory action research, which the authors have used to outline some principles for carrying this out. It is highly relevant, as it is based on working with people with mental health problems, although the lead comes from 'professional researchers' who are not identified as having mental health problems. However, it works to fully involve participants in the research process, and runs through issues such as training and support, power sharing and mutual respect, confidentiality and fluctuating participation.

It is quite common for the more formalised guidelines to be organised into categories of 'obligations', 'responsibilities' or 'accountabilities', in order to group the issues covered by the guidelines. For example, the Social Research Association (SRA), which in many ways is the most comprehensive, has five such categories:

- obligations to society;
- obligations to funders and employer;
- obligations to colleagues;
- obligations to subjects;
- ethics committees and Institutional Review Boards (US equivalent).

The British Sociological Association, which is less comprehensive but more 'user-friendly' in its language, has the following:

- professional integrity;
- relations with, and responsibilities towards, research participants;
- relations with, and responsibilities towards, research funders and sponsors.

Finally, the Mind/Trans-Cultural Psychiatry Society publication, *Getting the evidence: Guidelines for ethical mental health research involving issues of 'race', ethnicity and culture* (Patel, 1999) approaches it rather differently. Their overall focus tends to be at the 'community' level rather than at the individual level, which many of our topics tend to be. Many of their categories reflect the research timeline, but also – crucially – address the theoretical basis on which the research may be founded. Their categories are as follows:

- collaboration with communities studied;
- ideological and epistemological basis of research;
- formulating hypotheses;
- research design;
- data collection;
- data analysis;
- reporting results;
- discussion of findings;
- dissemination of research findings.

In developing the questionnaire and interview schedules for the current research, it was decided to group issues in a similar way to the SRA initially, looking at areas of responsibility and accountability. Although this worked in part, it was found that many people in individual and group interviews responded more easily to questions relating to the research process. Hence, the report guidelines follow a structure that is more similar to the Mind/ Trans-Cultural Psychiatry Society guidelines.

In Appendix B, the question is given in italics prior to the analysis of the results. These same question areas were used for the interviews and focus groups but with a less structured approach: in these situations, emphasis was placed on those areas in which the individual or group had the greatest experience.

Appendix B:
Analysis of questionnaires

Consultation questionnaire analysis

A total of 15 responses were received; 14 respondents identified themselves as service users/survivors, 13 as researchers, 11 as interviewers, nine as trainers, three as academics and six as mental health workers or professionals. One further wanted to identify as a human being and one as a committee member.

Underlying values or principles

Q. What underlying values or principles do you think should inform a set of guidelines for good practice in survivor research?

Tick one box if you think a topic should be included. Tick twice if you consider this topic to be particularly important.

User empowerment		
Equal opportunities		
Respect for all individuals involved in research		
The rights of participants and researchers		
Protection from harm		
Other (please state)		

This was an area of considerable consensus: all 15 people agreed that the following principles should be included:

- equal opportunities;
- respect for all individuals involved in research;
- the rights of participants and researchers.

Respect also had 10 votes for being 'particularly important', and equal opportunities had nine.

The other two principles (user empowerment and protection from harm) also received significant approval: 14 and 13 votes respectively.

A few additional values/principles were suggested: the importance of benefiting from taking part; that research be of good quality; the value of knowledge for its own sake; and the value of research as a tool for change.

Responsibilities to society

Q. Many guidelines for ethical research cover the need for the researcher or research community to be responsible in their activities to society at large. Please indicate below if you agree with any of these responsibilities in respect of society, and again add any you think need to be included.

Please tick one box if you think a topic should be included. Tick twice if you consider this topic to be particularly important.

Research to ...

... be socially inclusive and diverse (as is relevant to the research topic)		
... raise the profile of mental health/distress in society		
... counter stigma/discrimination based on mental illness diagnosis		
... be relevant to the wider society		
... be made available (disseminated) to relevant stakeholder communities		
Other (please state)		

This group of items received variable responses. Two received significant agreement, with 13 votes each for:

Research to ...

- counter stigma/discrimination based on mental illness diagnosis (seven voted this 'particularly important');
- be made available (disseminated) to relevant stakeholder communities.·

Others in this category received fewer votes (12, 11, 11) and one or two uncertain comments questioning the necessity for making user/survivor research relevant to the wider society.

Relations with, and responsibilities towards, mental health service users and survivors, groups and communities

Q. Do you believe that survivor research needs to have responsibilities towards relevant mental health service user groups, communities and individuals?

Yes	
No	
Not sure	

Some of the issues that might come under this heading are given below. Please indicate those that you think are important for good practice in survivor research.

Please tick one box if you think a topic should be included. Tick twice if you consider this topic to be particularly important.

Research topic to be of concern to the wider user/survivor community		
Researchers to make explicit any underlying beliefs or theories		
Research not to perpetuate stereotypes of people with mental health problems		
Research to be of high quality		
User and survivor communities to be free to use results of the research as they wish		
The impact of research to be meaningful to user/survivor groups and communities		
A commitment to implementing the results of research		
Results of research to be disseminated in accessible formats		
Other (please state)		

This was a particularly interesting category. Firstly, nine people responded positively to the question 'Do you believe that survivor research needs to have responsibilities towards relevant mental health service user groups, communities and individuals?'. Three responded 'No' and three 'Not sure'. In the following table, however, considerable consensus was reached on three of the eight items:

- the impact of research to be meaningful to user/survivor groups and communities (14/7);
- research not to perpetuate stereotypes of people with mental health problems (14/6);
- researchers to make explicit any underlying beliefs or theories (14/6).

A further two items also received some agreement:

- research to be of high quality (13/8);
- results of research to be disseminated in accessible formats (13/7).

Fewest votes (8/2) were given to the item 'Research topic to be of concern to the wider user/survivor community'.

In response to the item concerning implementing the results of research, some people expressed the doubt that survivor researchers would have the power or influence to ensure that this happened, although it may be a desirable ideal.

Relations with, and responsibilities towards, co-researchers, interviewers and trainees

Q. Researchers acting as 'project coordinators' or trainers, in particular, will have responsibilities to their co-researchers and interviewers, and to people they are training. The following options concern these relationships and responsibilities.

Please tick one box if you think a topic should be included. Tick twice if you consider this topic to be particularly important.

Respect, especially for people's right to differences of opinion	
Inclusivity: the principle that everyone can have a role in the research	
Support to be provided to all co-researchers and interviewers (eg debriefing)	
Training to be provided in relevant skills and other topics	
Pleasant training venue, refreshments, and time to get to know each other	
Clear personal supervision provided	
Confidentiality: the boundaries between interviewer and interviewee, and between co-researchers, to be respected	
Payment to be offered for all research work.... Advice and information made available about any impact on benefits	
Personal safety to be maximised; risk assessment to be made of the research endeavour	
Contact with Occupational Health departments to ensure ease of employment (where appropriate)	
Clarity about what to do if a co-researcher becomes 'unwell'	
A signed contract of commitment and expectations	
Other (please state)	

With the exception of the item on Occupational Health, which one or two people did not understand and others had no experience of, the items in this list received a fair amount of consensus. They are given next in descending order of votes:

14 votes:
- confidentiality: the boundaries between interviewer and interviewee, and between co-researchers, to be respected (10);
- support to be provided to all co-researchers and interviewers (eg debriefing) (8);
- training to be provided in relevant skills and other topics (8);
- respect, especially for people's right to differences of opinion (8);
- clarity about what to do if a co-researcher becomes 'unwell' (5);
- clear personal supervision provided (4).

13 votes:
- pleasant training venue, refreshments, and time to get to know each other.

12 votes:
- payment to be offered for all research work.... Advice and information made available about any impact on benefits (7);
- personal safety to be maximised; risk assessment to be made of the research endeavour (6);
- a signed contract of commitment and expectations (4).

11 votes:
- inclusivity: the principle that everyone can have a role in the research.

Several of these items provoked some interesting comments/debate. Two or three people felt that payment should not be seen as essential, particularly if the research coordinator is a service user/survivor without the resources to pay people. One person suggested that 'involved volunteers' should have a place in the process. The other side of this debate sees people feeling strongly that all people should be paid for carrying out work. However, it is possible that some people are influenced by their experience of research that is in the hands of academics or professionals who 'involve' service users, in which case payment is thought to be an essential part of that involvement.

The subject of inclusivity was also an interesting one. On the one hand, there are people who feel quite strongly that everyone who comes forward should be given a role in the research process. The other side of this argument is that the importance of achieving high quality research deems it necessary to be selective and recruit people on the basis of skills and experience, or merit.

Finally, one or two people commented that some of these items put considerable pressure on people; particularly, in this instance, the signed contract of commitment and expectations.

Relations with, and responsibilities towards, participants in the research

Q. Most guidelines for ethical research give this area the greatest emphasis. In any research we undertake, we need to give consideration to the well-being and dignity of the people who are being researched. Some of the options under consideration for this area are given below.

Please tick one box if you think a topic should be included. Tick twice if you consider this topic to be particularly important.

High quality of research, eg well-trained interviewers		
Confidentiality – and limits to confidentiality		
Informed consent, including accessible information		
Support in case of distress caused by participating in the research		
Maximise personal safety of participants		
Inclusion in research process (eg commenting on findings, draft reports)		
Payment for participating		
Complaints procedures to cover the experience of being involved as a participant		
Accessible feedback about the results of research, to include a copy of report		
Other (please state)		

In this section again, many items received significant agreement from respondents. One item, 'Informed consent', received 15 votes, and five items received 14 votes, in descending order as follows:

- confidentiality – and limits to confidentiality (9);
- high quality of research (8);
- accessible feedback about the results of research (7);
- support in case of distress caused by participating in the research (7);
- maximise personal safety of participants (5).

Two items received 13 votes:

- payment for participating;
- complaints procedures.

Lowest on the list was 'Inclusion in research process', which received 12 votes.

Working with/influencing research ethics committees

Q. Some research needs to get approval from a local Research Ethics Committee. This is usually research taking place within the context of existing services, where research participants (patients/service users) are currently in hospital or under the care of medical professionals.

Please tick one box if you think a topic should be included. Tick twice if you consider this topic to be particularly important.

Research Ethics Committees ...

... to spend time getting to know about user/survivor research, including examples of where users have been involved in research		
... to have more than one service user on the committee		
... to be more user-friendly to prospective applicants		
... to have established guidelines to ensure user views are heard and acted on		
... to give full feedback to applicants		
... to have a complaints procedure in place		
... to simplify the process of application		
... to have a clear confidentiality policy on members and applicants		
Other (please state)		

A couple of people said they had no experience of this and did not respond to this section; however, most people voted in favour of many of the items on the list. In order again, they are as follows:

13 votes:
- to simplify the process of application (9);
- to be more user-friendly to prospective applicants (8);
- to give full feedback to applicants (5);
- to have a clear confidentiality policy on members and applicants (5);
- to have a complaints procedure in place (3).

12 votes were awarded to the remaining items. An additional two items were proposed: quick decisions; and 'more appropriate to different types of research'.

In summary, these are the highest voted items in each category (14 or 15 votes):

Values/principles
- equal opportunities;
- respect for all individuals involved in research;
- rights of participants and researchers.

Responsibilities to participants
- informed consent;
- confidentiality, and limits to confidentiality;
- high quality of research;
- accessible feedback about the results of research;
- support in the case of distress caused by participating in the research;
- maximisation of personal safety of participants.

Responsibilities to co-researchers, interviewers and trainees
- confidentiality: the boundaries between interviewer and interviewee, and between co-researchers, to be respected;
- support to be provided to all co-researchers and interviewers (eg de-briefing);
- training to be provided in relevant skills and other topics;
- respect, especially for people's right to differences of opinion;
- clarity about what to do if a co-researcher becomes 'unwell';
- clear personal supervision provided.

Responsibilities to service user/survivor communities
- the impact of research to be meaningful to user/survivor groups and communities;
- research not to perpetuate stereotypes of people with mental health problems;
- researchers to make explicit any underlying beliefs or theories.

Ethics committees
None of these gained 14 or 15 votes; the highest at 13 were:

- to be more user-friendly to prospective applicants;
- to simplify the process of application.

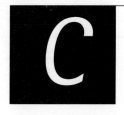

Appendix C:
Members of the advisory group

Peter Beresford
Professor of Social Policy and Director of the Centre for Citizen Participation, Brunel University, and Chair of Shaping Our Lives, the national user-controlled organisation

Andrew Hughes
Survivor Trainer, Researcher and Consultant; Mental Health Training and Distress Awareness Training Agency

Viv Lindow
Survivor Researcher/Consultant to the Project

Vicky Nicholls
Coordinator, Strategies for Living project; Mental Health Foundation

Debbie Tallis
Survivor Researcher

Premila Trivedi
Mental Health Service User